T0283853

Why Can't I See My GP?

Why Can't I See My GP?

The past, present and future
of general practice

Dr Ellen Welch

www.uwp.co.uk

British Library Cataloguing-in-Publication Data
A catalogue record for this book is available from the British Library.

ISBN: 978-1-915279-46-0

Cover artwork by Andy Ward
Typeset by Agnes Graves
Printed and bound by CPI Group (UK) Ltd, Croydon, CR0 4YY

Contents

Foreword

General practice is not the place it was when I first joined the profession almost 15 years ago. I used to enjoy going to work and seeing my patients; I rarely get that feeling now. It is in crisis. There is not a day that goes by without a story in the papers or online about people struggling to see their GPs. It is not because we as GPs are lazy fat cats hiding at home; it is because no matter how many patients we see, phone or consult with online, it will never be enough to keep up with demand. Despite the barrage of abuse we take from the media, we continue to go to work each day and try to do our best by our patients. There is a constant feeling of being on the back foot, and daily firefighting. But more than that, we know that because of the lack of investment in primary care over the years, there is a cohort of people out there who need to be seen and we simply do not have the capacity. As a result, somebody's serious health diagnosis is likely to be delayed, or worse, missed. This is an agonising thought.

It is a well-publicised fact that currently there are simply not enough GPs to deal with demand. It takes 10 years to train to be a GP: 5 years at medical school and then a further 5 years of postgraduate training. And that is only if they are training full time without gaps. I would argue that it takes another 5 years to gain the experience needed to become a confident GP. That's a long time. The job has become so difficult now that GPs are quitting or moving to countries where they feel more valued. New recruits are reluctant to work full time or commit to a single practice, because to do so risks burnout. Other healthcare professionals are being drafted in to plug the gaps.

But the problem is not simply a lack of capacity; it is also increasing demand. It is no secret we have an ageing population. Also, more and more services are being pushed out of hospital into the community, thereby increasing the demand put upon those of us working in primary care. On top of that, we have been through a pandemic, continue to pollute our air and waterways, have had a huge financial crisis and the cost of living has increased to levels previously unknown. All of these factors have an impact on the health of the population. Not a week goes by where I am not having to write a letter to support a patient in their application to get money off their energy bills, or bat off a request for a prescription for supplement drinks because someone cannot afford food. I have never had to do that before. As hospital lists get longer and longer, patients present back to their GPs with worsening symptoms, begging for medication to ease the pain or letters to speed up their hospital appointment dates.

Despite the increasing complexity of patients, the model of general practice has not changed much in decades. GPs still need to manage a patient within a 10- or 15-minute timeframe. And that time includes meticulously writing up notes (patients now have access to everything we write so our notes must be clear), doing any referrals and paperwork.

Improving primary care is going to take a multi-pronged approach. Yes, we need more GPs and investment in primary care services, but we also need to be clear about how we are going to tackle health inequalities and the social injustices that lead to poor health. It is a mammoth task, but we don't really have a choice. Primary care holds the NHS together; without us, the entire system collapses. Then what are we left with? A private healthcare system. Be under no illusion, we are fighting for our patients: their right to see a GP when they need to and to continue to receive health care free at the point of need. We are worth investing in.

Dr Amir Khan

Acknowledgements

This book is dedicated to Dr Gail Milligan, whose story you will read in chapter 3.

This book emerged from the work I was doing with the Doctors' Association UK and firstly I need to thank all of the wonderful team at DAUK, who voluntarily give up their free time to advocate for the profession, in particular Matt Kneale, Jenny Vaughan, Lizzie Toberty and Steve Taylor (whose knowledge of the facts and figures was invaluable in chapter 4). Big thanks also to Lucy, Sangeeta and Danny.

To my GP Twitter friends, who I've never even met in person, but have provided support and solidarity in supporting general practice over the past few years – Simon Hodes, Neena Jha, Shan Hussain, Ayan Panya, Selva Selvarajah and Dave Triska.

All the wonderful contributors to this book, who took the time to share their stories – thank you.

To James and Jess at Metro.co.uk, for giving us a platform and allowing us to reprint our opinion pieces here; and to Pulse and GPOnline reporters, who are great advocates for general practice.

Thanks to the Calon team, especially Abbie who was patient with me missing deadlines, and helped to bring order to the manuscript.

To the people in GP leadership positions who are making real steps towards change – huge thanks.

To my family, who have rallied round me during a personally difficult time and made me feel loved and supported – thank you.

We will all be patients one day, needing help from the NHS – and this book is an attempt to show what we have and why it is worth preserving. Thank you for reading.

Introduction

Dr Ellen Welch

I tried to contact my own GP last week. I counted 19 redials and 20 minutes on hold before I was able to speak to a receptionist…only to be told that all the appointments for the day had gone.

My experience echoes a familiar tale told up and down the country, but just why is it that you can't see your GP anymore?

This book provides some answers to that question.

In my case, I was given a telephone appointment with a GP in a fortnight, with no leeway given to negotiate further. As a GP myself, I know that when I speak to my own GP they are going to need to arrange a further face-to-face consult because an examination is needed… wasting a lot more time and appointments.

I've worked as a doctor for almost 20 years. I'd like to think I have an adequate understanding of how the NHS works, but my experience above illustrates that even GPs who work within the system day in day out can struggle accessing what they need as patients.

The reason you can't see your GP, and I can't see mine, doesn't really fit into a snappy soundbite. The data tells the story of just how hard the GP and wider NHS workforce have been toiling, but this workforce has been in decline since 2015. Funding has been static and NHS staff have had their pay frozen. When the Covid-19 pandemic hit in 2020, the NHS was already on the back foot after a decade of austerity. As I write this in 2023, the system is crumbling under the pressure.

Over recent years, NHS GPs have been working harder and harder to keep services afloat. Yet it feels like now more than ever, GPs have become the punchbag for a failing system. I wrote an article for GPonline for the 75th anniversary of the NHS[1] stating that despite still being proud of the job I do when it's done well, I avoid telling people I'm a GP. This is mainly because experience has told me that the response will often be either a rant about a terrible NHS experience, or well meaning, but misinformed comments about face-to-face appointments and GPs being closed throughout 2020. This book looks at where these ideas originate and explains the situation from the other side of the telephone queue – why GPs think it is difficult for patients to get seen. We hear from people who have spent their lives within the NHS observing the transformations that have occurred within the profession.

To give context to the present-day problems, we start with a brief history of general practice and how it formed within the NHS, and how things have changed to lead us to where we are today. NHS staff, supporters and patients share their personal stories, describing the changes experienced within their careers. Their accounts provide context to the NHS headlines we are fed each day and give insight into the current crisis within both general practice and the wider health service.

This isn't a book about me, but sharing my story may give some insight into why I've written this and why I feel so strongly that the voices of NHS staff need to be heard as part of a solution to the problems. I've been lucky enough to step off the NHS treadmill at different stages of my life, working as a doctor all over the world. I spent time as a junior doctor in New Zealand, including working a season as a ski field doctor in their Southern Alps. I did electives as a medical student in both Australia and Sri Lanka, gaining an understanding of how their health systems work. After training in emergency medicine in Yorkshire, I ran away to sea and started what would be a 10-year career as a cruise ship doctor. I didn't work in the countries we visited, but I liaised with their hospitals and clinics on an almost daily basis. So I have seen how health systems function outside of the UK. Occasionally in this role, when I saw people being handed hefty bills at the end of their treatment, I felt grateful to have the security of the NHS. I have also worked as a repatriation doctor, which involved helping people return home when they became ill overseas. And once again, some of the health care these people received made me deeply value the NHS.

I became a GP because of the experiences I had working on ships. The multinational crew, some of whom live on board for up to 9 months at a time, came to me with problems that I wouldn't typically deal with as an emergency medicine doctor, and it made me realise how much I valued the continuity of care – seeing people time and time again and sharing their journeys. I had never considered general practice as a career, but after two contracts at sea I applied for GP training back in the UK and returned to Cumbria to complete this.

Since then, I've worked as a GP in a tiny Lakeland practice, which at the time had less than 900 patients. I also spent several years in the heart of west London, in two much larger practices. I've done glorious home visits involving hiking through snow to remote cottages in the fells, and some terrifying ones in dark tower blocks in London. I've worked as an out-of-hours GP in both settings, and again, this has shown me just how different the job of a GP can be depending on the location, and why often the decisions made about GPs and the NHS from the government and NHS leaders, don't always translate to the daily reality on the ground.

This book brings together first-hand accounts from all over the country and overseas, from contributors with different working backgrounds and experiences, to try to distil the current feeling amongst the profession and to examine the reasons why our NHS has fallen from its pedestal.

In 2020, after returning from ships and starting a family in Cumbria, the pandemic hit. I was already working remotely for a national out-of-hours provider (so I could work but be close to my breastfed baby). I felt an enormous amount of guilt at this time, as colleagues faced the unknown – putting themselves at risk every shift with inadequate personal protective equipment (PPE), up against an unknown virus that was claiming lives. Thousands of healthcare staff died. We may remember the pandemic differently with hindsight now that the news agenda has moved on, but for the medical profession, who dealt stoically with the challenges, it was a traumatic time, and many staff are still suffering the effects. I can still recreate that cold feeling of dread that early 2020 brought, as we realised the NHS just wasn't prepared for the greatest public health challenge it had ever faced.

It was this guilt that prompted me to join the Doctors' Association UK (DAUK) in 2020, the guilt of working from home, instead of in 'the trenches' with my colleagues, balanced alongside the guilt of keeping my growing family safe (I was also pregnant at this time). This was misplaced guilt, I now realise. Motherhood is frantic in many new ways, but it did allow me to press the pause button when it came to work. My 'portfolio' career prior to motherhood was non-stop: always on the move, long shifts, keeping busy. Having babies was possibly harder than all that had come before, but the times when they slept in the early days, was time I used to campaign for DAUK.

DAUK's work is described in more detail at the end of this book. It is the work I've done alongside this fantastic group of people that opened my eyes to the corny, but true, fact that change comes from us all as individuals, and that change is multiplied when like-minded people work together. DAUK is composed of volunteer doctors, spending hours of their free time campaigning for the profession and the NHS, for free. The NHS is such a vast organisation, and inevitably it is led by fallible humans. Some of these leaders may never have set foot in a GP practice in their role, to understand the problems and hear from staff. Therefore, it is down to us to advocate for our profession – and ultimately our patients – and speak up about what is going on.

The media agenda has been led by politicians, and, for GPs in particular, the last few years have been brutal. Headlines have frequently contradicted what we know to be the day-to-day reality of the job. This book tells some of those stories, attempting to redress the balance. It allows you to hear the truth straight from the horse's mouth – why you can't see your GP. The final chapter of this book looks towards solutions, asks what needs to change and provides ways we can help as patients to preserve the future of UK general practice, so that we *can* see our GPs again.

Chapter 1
A brief history of NHS general practice

Ellie Philpotts with Dr Ellen Welch

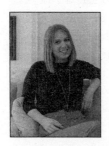

Ellie Philpotts is an award-winning health journalist, a teenage cancer survivor, charity campaigner and creative writer.

At midnight on 5 July 1948, medical care in the UK became free, based on a person's need rather than the ability to pay, and was available to all, including non-nationals living temporarily in Britain. Additional resources for the new NHS were negligible. The same number of doctors and nurses went to work in the same hospitals on the 5 July, the same way they had the day before. But what had changed, was improved accessibility for patients and a more equitable distribution of existing services. People who had delayed seeking help, sometimes for decades, were now able to be treated. The NHS was the first health system in the world to offer free care for all, and its founding principles were revolutionary.

So much has changed in the three quarters of a century since the creation of the NHS by Labour's Aneurin 'Nye' Bevan (see box below). This chapter touches on some milestones to give context to the state of general practice in 2023.

The twentieth century welcomed innovations in health care, such as the discovery of DNA; the first organ transplants and 'keyhole' surgeries; alongside the introduction of CT and MRI scanners. Milestones in women's rights and fertility were also achieved: the legalisation of abortion; widespread availability of the contraceptive pill; and later, IVF and 'test tube' babies. In the twentieth century, antipsychotic drugs transformed care for people with mental health problems, meaning that psychiatric care could be provided in the community.

Since the founding of the NHS, a huge culture shift has led to a society of expert patients who are healthcare consumers. General practice has had to adapt to the demands of an ageing population with multiple medical problems, a tightening of budgets, and the needs of patients who are more informed and accustomed to using technology for instant answers.

The founders of the NHS could not have anticipated these technological and cultural changes, which have led to it becoming the vast organisation it is today. It is now the fifth largest employer in the world and deals with 1.5 million patients every day – the equivalent of the entire population of Estonia.[2] Decades of reorganisations have shaped the service into the system we rely on today, and we have been raised with the expectation that health care will be available to us whenever we need it, without a bill. Regardless of our own upbringing, it has formed the background of our entire lives.

Aneurin 'Nye' Bevan

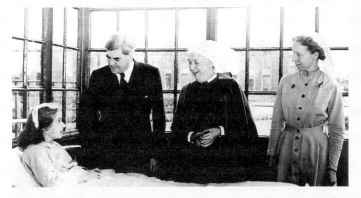

Aneurin 'Nye' Bevan (1897–1960) was the Labour Health Secretary credited with the creation of the NHS. A politician Wales was proud to call their own, Bevan was born in the south Wales mining community of Tredegar. Growing up, he was exposed to poverty and disease. Three out of his nine siblings died during childhood. His father was a coal miner, and Bevan followed suit, leaving school at age 13 to become a collier's helper. During that time, he became a trades union activist and won a scholarship to study in London. During the 1926 General Strike, he emerged as one of the leaders of the south Wales miners. In 1929, he went on to be elected as a Labour MP for Ebbw Vale. Bevan became well known as a champion for the working class, overcoming a speech impediment to become a passionate speaker.

Following Labour's landslide victory in 1945, he was appointed Minister for Health by Clement Attlee, and given the task of implementing the manifesto plans for a welfare state and healthcare revolution. Bevan recognised that health was a key factor in social inequality and made it his mission to tackle this issue head on.

As he launched the new NHS, he described it as 'the most civilised step any country has ever taken'.[3] He also rather prophetically said: 'I have been exhorting the general public to make use of this NHS prudently, intelligently and morally, because if too great a strain is placed upon it at the beginning it might break down. Because things are free is no reason why people should abuse their opportunity.'[4]

During planning, the predicted annual cost of the NHS was £170 million. However, demand for the service exceeded all predictions. In its first full year of operation, costs exceeded £305 million. Spectacle prescriptions alone had produced a bill amounting to £32 million, when the budget had been £1 million.

In 1950, Hugh Gaitskell became Chancellor of the Exchequer. He proposed that annual savings of £13 million could be made by imposing charges for dentures and spectacles provided by the NHS. Bevan resigned from government the very next day in protest, unwilling to compromise his free-at-the-point-of-use ideals. The Conservative government went on to introduce charges for prescriptions of 1 shilling (5p) in 1952. A prescription in 2023 costs £9.35 per item.

Bevan continued as a Labour backbencher, running unsuccessfully for leadership of the party in 1955. He became Deputy Leader in 1959, but died of cancer in 1960, leaving behind a legacy as the father of the NHS.

The birth of general practice

General practice is the biggest medical speciality within the NHS, with 36,488 fully qualified GPs working in the NHS in England in January

2023.[5] Back in 1952, when this data was first available, there were only 17,204 GPs in both England and Wales. Although its 'cradle to grave' tradition isn't now as feasible as it once was, most people still have access to a GP to see them through life's ills.

It hasn't always been this way. Prior to the creation of the NHS, GPs worked as independent traders, treating people who had the money to pay them, often from a consulting room in their own home. At the turn of the twentieth century, conditions were harsh. In a time before vaccines and antibiotics, annual death rates for diseases such as tuberculosis, diphtheria, meningitis and pneumonia ran into their thousands; industrial diseases were rife and one in 20 children died before their first birthday.[6]

The early seeds of a universal NHS were sown in 1911, when Prime Minister David Lloyd George issued his National Insurance Act, which provided the UK working classes with a contributory national insurance scheme. Lloyd George's Act provided the assurance of basic medical care from a GP to working men during periods of illness, as long as they paid their compulsory insurance contributions to the scheme. It aimed to relieve hardship among the working classes and avoid them seeking help from the stigmatised provisions of the Poor Law and the workhouses. Paying workers were given access to free treatment from a panel doctor (a GP) of their choosing; however, their wives and families weren't covered by this system and hospital care was not funded, so many men resented giving up their hard-earned wages for the scheme, and many people continued to experience hardship.

Life before the NHS

RAF Veteran Harry Leslie Smith, who died in 2018, grew up in poverty in Barnsley in the 1920s. Until his death, he frequently spoke in support of the NHS, describing how common preventable diseases 'snuffed out life like a cold breath on a warm candle flame' prior to the creation of the service. His sister caught tuberculosis at a young age, which infected her spine and left her bedbound by the age of 10. As Harry's family were unable to care for her, his sister was sent to the neighbourhood workhouse, which housed prisoners, sick paupers and the mentally ill. She died there soon afterwards. 'I will never forget, as long as I shall live,' said Smith, 'the screams that fell out of dosshouse windows from the dying and mentally ill, who were denied medicine and solace because they didn't have the money to pay for medical services.'[7]

The framework for the NHS, however, grew from Lloyd George's Act. It created the idea of state-funded medical care for lists of registered patients and the principle of capitation payments to GPs for patients on their panels. It formalised the practice of referrals from GPs to hospital specialists, launching the role of a GP as a gatekeeper to secondary care.

In 1920, a report from military physician Lord Bertrand Dawson was commissioned by the recently formed Ministry of Health, aiming to link hospitals into a single system available to all citizens. This report laid the blueprint for the NHS, which was launched 30 years later.[8]

The report described a service model consisting of primary health centres which could include additional resources for GPs alongside their own consulting rooms, such as laboratory tests and radiology, and it envisaged GPs working together in groups rather than alone (to much protest from the profession). Secondary health centres, or hospitals, would manage specific conditions, operating within districts, while university hospitals would provide the most specialised services. The report recognised the need for an administrative hierarchy, and outlined health authorities, with control of curative and preventative services.

Dawson's proposals were backed several years later by a report from the Royal Commission on National Health Insurance, which advocated for medical services to be divorced entirely from the insurance system, in the same way as public health services, and funded by the general public. In 1930, the British Medical Association (BMA) agreed that health insurance coverage should be given to the whole population, and that a coordinated regional hospital service should be instituted. Over the next decade, depression and economy cuts dominated, which destroyed any chance of significant reform.

The impact of war

The year 1939 brought the start of the Second World War, which hugely disrupted life for everyone across the country, including the healthcare system. A national Emergency Medical Service (EMS) was set up to care for civilians injured during air raids, and doctors and nurses were paid by the state to treat patients in voluntary hospitals.

The war changed attitudes. The state controlled most aspects of people's lives during this period, often with good outcomes. Rationing improved the health of the poor, and the EMS response to treating casualties gave people access to health care that they had never experienced before.

In 1942, economist Sir William Beveridge chaired the committee tasked with reviewing social insurance schemes. The resulting 'Report on Social Insurance and Allied Services' became more succinctly known as 'The Beveridge Report'. This report set out plans for the future of post-war Britain and laid the foundation for the modern welfare state. It called for a solution for the 'five giant evils' that blighted the lives of British people: want, disease, ignorance, squalor and idleness, and proposed a state-operated system of social security to include a national health service. It suggested that all working people should pay a contribution to a state fund that could be used for a comprehensive health service, the avoidance of mass unemployment and a system of children's allowances.

The white paper, 'A National Health Service', was published by Conservative Sir Henry Willink in 1944. It outlined the wartime coalition government's vision for a free, unified health service. It proposed central government management, with responsibility for its provision lying with the minister for health. The minister ultimately appointed to this position in 1945 was Labour's Aneurin Bevan, whose proposals for the service went further than what had been discussed before. Bevan was adamant that funding should come primarily from taxation rather than National Insurance, and that it must be available free for all.

His intention was also to make all doctors salaried employees of the NHS – an idea that in 1920 the Dawson Report had flagged as bad news for patients. Private practice was to be banned within the nationalised hospitals, although an agreement was reached where specialist doctors could reduce their time contracted to the NHS to give them time to undertake private practice, with a small number of private beds allocated to accommodate this. GPs were to be treated differently. As self-employed practitioners, they traditionally sold their practices on retirement and used the goodwill capital (goodwill being the money raised when a business is sold at a price greater than the value of its assets) to fund their pensions. GPs insisted on remaining independent contractors, arguing that they needed to be advocates for their patients within a state-run system. This came to pass, the compromise being that the sale of goodwill was outlawed, and GPs became eligible to use the NHS pension scheme instead.

The new NHS

In 1948, the NHS was divided into three parts:

- Hospital services managed by 400 hospital management committees, under the control of 14 regional hospital boards.
- Community services (i.e. midwifery and health visiting services, school medical services, ambulance services, immunisation and public health) which remained the responsibility of the local authorities.
- Primary care (GPs, dentists, opticians and pharmacists) which were to be independent contractors to the NHS.

GPs were contracted to the NHS to provide all necessary care for a defined list of patients. They remained free to organise their own practices, but NHS work was controlled by a tightly defined contract, nationally negotiated between the BMA and the government. The Spens Report determined pay, which was entirely by capitation, meaning GPs received a fee for each patient registered with them. Their expenses were averaged and included in the payment-per-patient. No money could pass directly between patient and doctor (with few exceptions such as payment for a private medical certificate). This arrangement meant GPs were taxed as though they were self-employed, but they could not set their own fees in the same way most small businesses can. This removed any financial incentives to overtreat patients, but also meant any improvements made to services had no financial reward attached.[9]

The impact of the NHS on doctors and patients

In 1947, Dr John Fry opened his single-handed practice in Beckenham. A year later, he became an independent contractor in the NHS, free to work as he judged appropriate, within the terms of his contract.

I worked from the same premises as before with the same arrangements for consultations and home visits for the same patients and with the same part-time staff, my wife. Nevertheless, there were great differences. No longer did my patients have to pay or feel inhibited from seeking any help because of cost, nor did I have to worry how much to charge and whether I would be paid. No longer did my wife and I have to spend midnight hours sending out monthly accounts, of which one in five were never paid. No longer did I have to dispense medicines or worry whether the patient could afford the more expensive ones, I merely wrote a 'free' NHS prescription for what I thought was appropriate. No longer was there any distinction between 'private patients' and the less privileged 'panel patients', for all NHS patients carried the same annual capitation fee. It was real democracy at work.

In my Beckenham practice, there was no immediate change in the nature or volume of work. However, nationally, the first effect of the NHS was mass euphoria, the second was of massive demands of hitherto unmet social and medical needs. There was a rush for 'free' spectacles, dentures and hearing aids, and the work of hospitals and general practitioners (GPs) increased. Amazingly, the new NHS coped with these demands reasonably well, because of the tolerance and goodwill of public and profession alike. Yet it soon became clear that a huge medical industry had been taken over but with no administrative and organisational arrangements to promote effectiveness, efficiency and economy. [10]

Lord Beveridge had predicted that the initial jump in demand for GP services would eventually fall, but this never happened, and GPs were overwhelmed with demands from patients who had for financial reasons previously avoided seeking care. Within a month of the creation of the NHS, 90 per cent of the population registered with a GP.[11] Each GP was personally responsible for the care of their patients 24 hours a day, 7 days a week, 365 days a year, meaning single-handed doctors (the term for GPs running their practices alone, without other GP partners) could be on call round the clock with no respite.

Gone

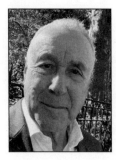

Roy Lilley is a health policy analyst, writer, broadcaster and commentator on health care. This piece first appeared on his blog. [12]

The boy had been ill for a couple of days. Neither mum, nor grandma knew what to do. This was different.

The new NHS was supposed to be free. Few working people really believed it.

A doctor's visits cost half a crown. Half a crown more than the family of a window cleaner could find.

It was 10 o'clock in the evening when dad decided something had to be done. 'If it's free,' he said, 'we'll find out.'

He wrapped the boy in a blanket and walked the mile, through narrow terraced streets, across the high street, underneath the railway arches, to where the streets widened into an avenue…

…the pavements were lined with trees. 'The doctor's was a two storey, elegant, detached house with a veranda at the front, a manicured lawn and driveway.

The lights were on in an upstairs room.

The man closed the gate, quietly, behind him. His footsteps crunching on the gravel. He pulled at the bell, heard it jangle somewhere in the distance and waited.

The hall lights came on, bolts slid across…a man in a dressing-gown opened the door.

The man, with the boy in his arms, said, 'Doctor, I know it's late… we didn't know what to do, it's my lad he's very poorly…his mum's worried sick.'

The doctor smiled and waved the man along the hallway, to the downstairs room that was his surgery.

Most doctors at that time worked from home. And, like many, this doctor's wife was a nurse, arranged the house calls, did the paperwork and changed the dressings.

The examination was over in minutes. As the doctor washed his hands, in the sink in the corner of the room, he said: 'He's not well at all. He needs to go to hospital.'

The man searched for the words; how would he get there, what would it cost…

The doctor said: 'Don't worry. It'll be alright. We'll go in my car. We can try out Mr Bevan's new NHS.'

The Humber, with its walnut dashboard, smelt of leather. It was the first time the man had been in a private car.

The boy had a bowel obstruction and survived. The treatment was free, and Doctor Brown would, once a month, have his windows cleaned, with the compliments of the grateful dad.

I was that boy, and the dad was my dad, and…

…Dr Brown wore a waistcoat, we wore the jumpers my mum knitted. The Doc had cuff-links, we rolled up our sleeves. He had a car, we had bikes…but he was one of us, one of the community, and we loved him. When he died, pretty well all his patients turned out for the funeral.

Those days are gone. Family practice has given way to industrialised primary care.

Is it better…dunno. But what I do know is…

…the icy, winds of change are howling from the east. The war in Ukraine has triggered rising costs that few families will cope with, no governments are prepared for, and some GP practices will be lucky to survive.

We get 90 per cent of first contacts in care from GPs. They are paid less than 11 per cent of the NHS budget.

Practices are businesses. Like any other business, if they can't cover their costs…what's the point. Practices are facing a battering from inflation in the cost of consumables and specialist supplies running at around 15 per cent. They have to pay a 4.5 per cent uplift in pay, for Agenda for Change clinicians working in the practice, and it is not funded from the centre. Fuel costs are not capped for businesses; and like everyone else, they'll struggle to pay the bills.

Other staff, receptionists, admin, cleaners and others, just like everyone else, will have to take home more money. If they can't, they'll take themselves somewhere they can.

GP partners, like any other small business proprietor, will ask themselves: is it worth the pressure, responsibility, the oppression from NHS England, the criticisms, demands and expectations?

They can hand back their contract, become a locum, work as and when they want, earn no-less, without all the hassle.

The government has no answer, neither NHS England nor the Department of Health, because there is no answer.

Once, like my dad, we reached out a hand for help. Mistakenly, we came to think we could click our fingers and demand it...

...soon we'll look through the spaces between our fingers and wonder where it's gone.

Standards of care

The early years of the NHS saw GPs overwhelmed with demands from patients. In 1953, it was estimated that GPs were making between 12 and 30 home visits each day, as well as seeing between 15 and 50 patients in their surgeries.[13] Working hours had no boundaries, leading to many doctors working round the clock, impacting their morale and their standards.

This quote from 1950, reflecting the morale of GPs at the time, could just as easily have been written today.

The doctor is irritable with the patients and they are noticing it and commenting on it. The patients are more aggravating and the doctor is noticing it. GPs had been promised more help, an easier life and no bad debts. He had got much more work, in some cases less income as private practice slumped.

*The patients had a hospital service which, save in an emergency, they could only use by appointment after a wait of several weeks; and a free GP service rushed to the point of indecency. His haemorrhoids had to bleed for **six** months before he could be treated; her heavy periods for nine months before she could get a hysterectomy. And having been in hospital the patient could be home two weeks before the GP got a report.[14]*

The infamous Collings Report of 1950[15] was the first major report on quality in general practice. Its author, Joseph Collings, an Australian GP, described 'dirty and ill-equipped' consulting rooms with 'rusty and dusty antique instruments' and doctors who doled out sickness certificates and bottles of medicine on demand. He concluded that the 'overall state of general practice is bad and still deteriorating' and for inner city practice, 'at best…very unsatisfactory and at worst a positive source of public danger'. He noted that GPs were constantly being asked to do more work for less pay and recognised that it was in the interests of the government to invest in general practice to reduce the burden on expensive hospitals. He ended saying: 'If the present trend continues, it must result in the elimination of general practice as an effective agency of medical care.'

The report caused waves throughout the profession, triggering reflection by some GPs. Concerned about the reputation of their profession, a group of GPs founded the College of General Practitioners in November 1952, an academic body to guide GPs to improve standards and to establish general practice as a discipline. That same year, GPs also received a large, backdated pay increase to encourage new doctors to enter practice and form partnerships and group practices. This was called the Danckwerts Award.[16]

The college was granted its Royal Charter in 1972, becoming the Royal College of General Practitioners (RCGP). It has had a lasting impact on education and training ever since. In 1976, parliament approved legislation requiring doctors who wanted to become principals in general practice to complete vocational training, and of course even today, completion of the RCGP membership exams is a prerequisite for entering the profession.

There has been much debate over the years about the title of 'GP' and whether we need to rename ourselves as 'consultant family physicians' or similar. Outside the UK, many countries denote the title 'general practitioner' to any doctor who has finished their basic training but is yet to start specialty training. In the UK we undertake specialist training in being a generalist and perhaps recognition of this would give the profession a boost. When general practice took shape in the late nineteenth century, GPs were considered inferior to their hospital colleagues. Dr Julian Tudor-Hart described GPs as 'men who failed to become specialists and were unable to work in a hospital or to use its resources without going through their consultant colleagues'.[17] This legacy lingers on in the minds of the public and our colleagues, evident from questions such as 'When are you going to specialise?' to longstanding GPs, or requests from patients to bypass us and be directly referred to 'the specialist' for problems that GPs manage every day.

Consultants are defined as experts, so creating a GP 'consultant' role could reinvigorate general practice by proclaiming that we, as GPs, are expert medical generalists. GP leaders at the 2023 UK London Medical Council (LMC) conference in London backed a motion to recognise the key role of GPs in delivering continuity of care and leading multidisciplinary teams, backing calls to rebrand them as consultants in family medicine.[18]

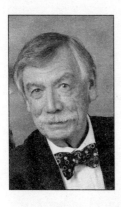

The history of out-of-hours GP services

Dr Eric Rose was an NHS GP for 36 years. From 1989 until 2008, he was a member of the GP Committee of the BMA and played a leading role in the campaign to reform GP out of hours. This piece has been adapted from a blog Dr Rose first wrote in 2013.[19]

The early days of the NHS

Before 1948, general practice was a cottage industry. Most GPs worked independently, usually from a consulting room in their own house. There were few, if any, staff, with the duties of answering the phone usually falling to the GP's wife (most doctors were at that time male) or, in some cases, a housekeeper, like the indomitable Janet of *Dr Finlay's Casebook*.

When the NHS was created, GPs feared the idea of becoming salaried employees of the state and held out against it. Eventually a compromise deal was reached in which GPs would work for the NHS but as independent contractors rather than employees. (It is worth mentioning, as it is often forgotten, that dentists, pharmacists and opticians also carry out NHS work as independent contractors.)

Much of the independence of GPs was, however, illusory. Whilst they remained free to organise their own practices, the work they did for the NHS was controlled by a very tightly defined contract.

A framework already existed; Lloyd George's National Insurance Act of 1911 provided for limited health cover for working men (but not their families). The scheme was administered by local insurance committees, covering counties and large conurbations, which held a list or panel of doctors prepared to work under the scheme. The panel doctors were subject to extensive 'terms of service' which were later lifted directly into the NHS GP contract.

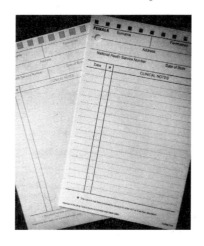

The NHS also adopted the medical record system used by local insurance committees. Known colloquially as 'Lloyd George records' they consisted of cards contained in a card envelope, which were still in widespread use nearly 100 years later.

1948 onwards
GPs' 24-hour responsibility

Over the years, the name and form of the local body responsible for administering family doctor services changed several times and the terms of service embellished. The main clauses however, remained unaltered. Two of which are most significant. Firstly, the contract was an individual one. That is to say that virtually every doctor working in general practice had a personal contract with the local NHS body and patients were registered with a named doctor. Salaried GPs or assistants were a rarity. Secondly, there was a clause which stated: 'A doctor is responsible for ensuring the provision for his patients of the services referred to…throughout each day during which his name is included in the…medical list.' This meant that each GP was personally responsible for the care of their patients 24 hours a day 7 days a week and 365 days a year. Any failure in that provision could result in the GP being hauled before the dreaded Medical Service Committee and a 'withholding of remuneration' or fines.

For single-handed doctors this meant being on call to patients round the clock with no respite, unless they could find a locum, which was not easy. Even for those in partnership it meant a gruelling on duty rota. As well as the doctor himself (most doctors were at that time male), the family were involved, as at nights and weekends GPs were on call from home with no other provision for answering the telephone.

1966 – Family Doctor Charter

By the early 1960s, working conditions were such that there was a major recruitment crisis in general practice, with many newly qualified doctors preferring to work in Australia or Canada rather than for the NHS. The then Health Secretary agreed to the 1966 Family Doctor Charter – a new contract and system of payment which provided, amongst other things, access to funding for new surgery buildings and partial reimbursement of wages for ancillary staff. It also included a 'group practice allowance' to encourage GPs to work together in practices.

Despite this, individual contracts and personal round-the-clock responsibility remained.

Group practices provided some respite as it was possible for the doctors to take it in turns to cover the out-of-hours period when the surgery was closed. However, since the average partnership size was only four or five doctors, this still meant around one night a week and one weekend a month, or more if a partner was away on holiday. This was in addition to daytime work in the surgery.

In some large cities, commercial deputising services were set up, employing doctors to cover the out-of-hours period, but these weren't viable in much of the country. Their use was also often limited by the local Family Practitioner Committee to a fixed number of calls, and frowned on by many politicians who felt that some GPs were being paid for staying in bed. The fact that these doctors had to give up part of their own income to pay the deputising company was either not understood or glossed over.

Personal experience

My own experience was that I entered general practice in 1972, choosing deliberately to go to an area which wasn't covered by a deputising service as I felt I wanted to give complete care to the patients in my practice. At first, as I was only 28 and came from working a hospital rota of one in two (which means being 'on call' for emergencies every other day), the work seemed manageable. Sometimes if I had been up in the night, there was an hour between morning and evening surgeries to take a nap. I actually enjoyed some night calls, especially in the summer. Going out and being able to relieve pain or help someone with breathing problems could be a pleasure, although it didn't stop me from being tired the next day.

Over the next few years, however, things began to change. Daytime surgeries got busier and the gap in the middle of the day disappeared. Although most patients were reasonable, an increasing minority regarded it as their right to ask the doctor to visit in the evening regardless of whether it was an emergency; some names cropped up so regularly that they were suspected of deliberately waiting till the surgery was closed before asking as they were then more likely to get a home visit. Some even thought they were calling a special night service instead of their own doctor who had already been working all day.

Family life had to be planned around the on-call rota; my wife, who by now had her own job, had to be home by 6pm to answer the phone, and during my weekends on call, couldn't leave the house at all. The children were also restricted; it was only when my son was in his forties that he told me how my weekends on call had upset him. I was on call and unable to visit my wife in hospital after our second child was born and was also on call when my older son had a serious accident at home. I remember kneeling beside him trying to staunch bleeding with one hand whilst holding the phone in the other trying to find someone to cover my duty.

My social life also suffered as non-medical friends couldn't understand why we couldn't join in all of their activities. Even when it was possible to go, I soon established a reputation for falling asleep at the dinner table due to having been up all night before.

In my practice, weekends on duty began at 9am on Friday and lasted until Monday evening. During the week before, I would become increasingly tense, and by the Monday night I was usually so stressed that relaxation came only from a bottle.

One additional factor that no-one seemed to consider is that GPs answering night calls to patient's homes had to drive themselves, often whilst in an exhausted state. As I turned 40, the thought of continuing to work like this for the next 25 years filled me with horror. But there seemed little likelihood of change, and I remember being treated as an oddity by senior colleagues at a regional RCGPs meeting when I said that I thought we should work to change the contract.

The 1990s – GP opinion changes

Gradually it became apparent that I was not alone in my beliefs, and there were also other forces at work. There were an increasing number of women entering general practice and they often needed to juggle family commitments around on-call duties. What childcare facilities there were in the NHS ceased to operate outside 'normal' working hours. Spouses of both male, and now female GPs had careers of their own and couldn't be at home as an unpaid telephone answerer.

The workload continued to rise and Health Secretary Kenneth Clarke's imposition of a new and more demanding contract in 1990 made many doctors feel that the trade-off of 24-hour responsibility for independence was increasingly unattractive. A BMA survey showed that an overwhelming majority of GPs at this time wanted to be relieved of the 24-hour contract. In 1992 the BMA began a campaign to get rid of the contractual obligation, which made GPs themselves responsible for organising and providing a round-the-clock service.

We adopted the slogan 'tired doctors are not good doctors'. Surprisingly, the press was largely sympathetic and understood that GPs couldn't go on working all hours. As so often happens, politicians refused to listen to the arguments, with ministers claiming that most of the time GPs were on call they were comfortably at home with their families. They were in any case, it was stated, paid a generous fee for night visits. This fee was not a bonus, it came out of the overall envelope allocated for GP remuneration. It was only paid for home visits after 10pm, which could amount to only a handful each month. This ignored the fact that the greatest burden of out-of-hours work was in the evenings and weekends. On a single Sunday at around this time I was called out 37 times and this was by no means uncommon. Only two of those calls qualified for these payments, which were, in any case, only payable to GPs working in small rotas of fewer than 10 doctors. The GP payment system was, and still is, complex, but the total amount earmarked for out-of-hours duties, including night-visit fees, was an average of just under £6,000 per GP per year.

1996 – GP out-of-hours cooperatives

Around 1994, the Department of Health organised a meeting of family health service managers from around the country. They wanted to brief them on the government line on maintaining the 24-hour contract. But they were in for a shock, as instead, many of the managers, who at that time had a close knowledge of the GPs in their area, reported that their local GPs were on their knees and the system was unsustainable.

When Stephen Dorrell became Health Secretary, he vowed to resolve the dispute. What he produced were some small changes in the wording of the contract. This, firstly, made it clear that GPs did not have to respond to every request for a home visit, but, where clinically appropriate, could see patients at their premises. Secondly, it stated that the full night-visit fee could be paid to doctors working in larger rotas. In addition, Dorrell set up an out-of-hours development fund, which would pay out an average of £3,000 per GP to support and encourage new ways of working.

The response of GPs was immediate and massive. All over the country, groups got together to form out-of-hours cooperatives: organisations which shared the out-of-hours work between a large number of local GPs. Within months, premises were found and staff, such as receptionists and drivers, were employed. Some cooperatives employed nurses with enhanced training to triage calls, but the medical work still had to be done by local doctors themselves. In some cases, this work was on a compulsory rota, while in others it was possible for the doctor to buy out of their shifts and pay others to do the work. But the bottom line remained: GPs still had round-the-clock individual responsibility for the provision of a service to their patients. If the cooperative collapsed or if not enough doctors were willing to do their shifts, then the responsibility fell to GPs to cover their own out-of-hours work.

Experience showed that a minimum of around 40 GPs were needed to set up a successful cooperative. This was relatively easy when based on a large town. But against all the odds, they were also made to work in more rural areas such as Cornwall.

But not every GP was part of one of these groups; in remote areas where a cooperative was not possible, GPs continued to be responsible for providing round-the-clock cover. A few practices decided they would prefer to cover their own patients and the commercial deputising companies continued to operate in large conurbations.

2000 – The Carson Report

Largely, patients took to the new system which meant that, instead of getting a home visit from their own doctor or a partner, they would, unless bedbound, be seen at a special out-of-hours surgery. In some cases, this meant travelling to a nearby town. Inevitably, there were complaints about this which were taken up vociferously by local MPs. At the same time, there were some reports by the health service ombudsman of problems, mainly involving commercial deputising services. One complaint involving a commercial deputising service for which I was an advisor to the ombudsman, involved insufficient doctors being employed and a 7-hour delay in seeing a seriously ill patient who later died.

As a result of these concerns, the Department of Health commissioned a team under Dr David Carson to investigate all GP out-of-hours services. The Carson Report,[20] published in 2000, proposed some stringent quality standards and made it clear that the standards should apply, not only to organisations such as deputising services and GP cooperatives, but also to individual GPs and practices still providing their own cover.

Carson also proposed: 'A new model of integrated out-of-hours provision should be accessed by patients via a single telephone call, routed in the first place through NHS Direct and passed, where necessary, to the appropriate provider of out-of-hours services in that locality.'

However, one of the basic premises stated by Carson was that: 'The provision of family doctor services will continue to be based on the patient list system, with GPs retaining 24-hour responsibility for their list.'

Paradoxically, the report also said: 'The Primary Care Trust will have overall responsibility for the planning of out-of-hour services in its locality…all out-of-hours services in a given locality (including GP out-of-hours services, A&E, ambulance and NHS Direct) should be planned as a single integrated service'.

It is clear that the ministers of the time and the Department of Health were enamoured by this idea, as a subsequent report of the Health Select Committee was to reveal.

The 2004 GP contract

By the start of the 2000s, for several reasons, GP morale was at an all-time low. Recruitment was increasingly difficult. In the 1980s, an advertisement for a partner might have brought in as many as 80 well qualified applicants; by the year 2000, there would rarely be more than a handful of applicants. Some practices received no applicants at all, leaving the existing partners to cope with an ever-increasing workload.

As discussed earlier, GPs never received a salary from the NHS; instead, there was a complex system of fees and allowances, leaving a GP's personal income to be derived from what was left after paying the running costs of the surgery.

In a national ballot at this time, GPs overwhelmingly voted for a new contract. At the same time, under the influence of Downing Street advisors, the Labour government had its own agenda, including opening-up primary care to a wider variety of providers and introducing a form of performance-related pay.

The mythology around the 2004 GP contract is that the BMA dictated the terms and the NHS employers team who represented the government were a soft touch, resulting in a contract which paid GPs a lot more for doing less work. The reality is that while negotiations were conducted in a spirit of cooperation, they were very detailed. There were many long meetings over a period of nearly 2 years. The Department of Health, the Treasury and Downing Street advisors were present every step of the way and they reported everything back to their ministers. The final contract was signed off by then Health Secretary, John Reid, who was not a pushover. Indeed, when some GPs expressed anxieties about agreeing to the new GP contract the attitude of Reid was one of 'no renegotiation'.

2004 – Responsibility for organising out-of-hours passes to primary care trusts (PCTs)

With regard to the out-of-hours part of the contract, the BMA was clear that the model of individual GPs having total responsibility both for organising and providing round-the-clock cover was unsustainable. The Department of Health was attracted to the idea of an integration of out-of-hours care as recommended by the 2000 Carson Report, which they thought would not only be better for patients but would help reduce costs.

As a subsequent report of the Health Select Committee stated:

Although there were differences of opinion on many issues relating to GP out-of-hours services, our witnesses gave a clear and unanimous message that the handover of responsibility for GP out-of-hours services from GPs to PCTs represented an excellent opportunity to redesign out-of-hours provision for the better, designing services around patients and developing a new model of primary out-of-hours care that dovetailed with the wider economy of unscheduled care provision, including A&E departments, ambulance services, GP emergency clinics, Walk-In Centres, NHS Direct, and local authority social services provision. [21]

So, the clause in the new contract, which allowed GPs to opt out of their total 24/7/365 responsibility, clearly suited both sides. It must be stressed that this did not abolish the out-of-hours GP service, it merely passed the responsibility for organising it from individual doctors to the primary care trusts (PCTs). As for the cost to individual GPs of giving up the 24-hour responsibility, much has been made of a subsequent television programme in which one of the eight BMA GP negotiators expressed surprise that it was only £6,000. But this figure wasn't plucked out of the air; it equated exactly to that part of GP ' pre-2004 income, which had been earmarked for out-of-hours work.

As well as this £6,000 per GP figure, PCTs would have access to the average £3,000 per GP in the out-of-hours development fund. In other words, they had exactly the same amount of money that GPs had used to fund the very successful out-of-hours cooperatives.

In less than 10 years, the GP cooperatives had built up a great deal of expertise in organising out-of-hours cover and their management boards comprised local GPs. It might be supposed that PCTs would automatically want to use this expertise.

But this was not the case. The NHS Confederation (the managers own organisation) told the Health Select Committee that few PCTs were working positively with GP cooperatives, often instead being adversarial and generating conflict. In Buckinghamshire, the GP cooperative was forced out of business, literally overnight, when the PCTs awarded the contract to a large company called Harmoni. In Cornwall, the exemplary KernowDoc was passed over in favour of a commercial company, Serco. Both Harmoni and Serco were later the subject of major complaints and, in particular, have been accused of failing to employ sufficient doctors. Ironically, these cases mirror the very situation which led to the 2000 Carson Report. Despite these experiences, a bid led by a group of East London GPs to take back organisation of out-of-hours care for their patients, was passed over in favour of a private company.

It is clear that the responsibility for any failings and shortcomings in out-of-hours GP services should rest not with GPs but with the PCTs, which were, until 1 April 2013, responsible for arranging the service. As long ago as 2004, the Health Select Committee recognised the risks and warned that many PCTs had failed fully to consider the risks, and the responsibility for organising these services was often being handled at a junior level. Clearly, in many cases this warning was not heeded.

Are GPs working less?

With regard to the rest of GPs' work, there is no doubt that the 2004 contract delivered a very welcome funding increase to practices and, therefore, an increase in GPs' personal income, but in the intervening 19 years this has been steadily eroded as funding levels have not kept pace with inflation and the increasing population, whilst the running costs of surgeries and staff pay have increased. In addition, the Department of Health has year on year increased the work that has to be done in order to qualify for payments. Despite being relieved of the round-the-clock responsibility, most GPs are working hours well above the national average.

It is clear that there has been a steady increase in the number of GPs working part time, which is not surprising considering that over 50 per cent of entrants are now women, who, as in other walks of life, are likely to want to work part time for at least part of their careers. The clinical work of GPs has also expanded; they are now expected to manage many conditions, which were in the past dealt with in hospital, and available treatments and investigations have increased exponentially. To give just one example, when I was a junior hospital doctor in the late 1960s, patients who suffered a myocardial infarction (heart attack) were kept in hospital for 6 weeks. Now, they are often diagnosed, treated and discharged within hours.

GPs also have an increasing amount of non-clinical work. As well as carrying ultimate responsibility for running their own practices, they may be involved in teaching trainees, in the appraisal of existing GPs and involved in local bodies running the health service.

How GP out-of-hours care changed

- Prior to 2004, GPs were working to a 90-year-old contract clause which made them personally responsible for providing round-the-clock services.
- By the turn of the century, this had become unsustainable.
- The Department of Health had an agenda to integrate out-of-hours services.
- The 2004 GP contract passed the responsibility for organising out-of-hours GP services from individual GPs to PCTs.

- The amount of money given up by GPs equated to what they received for out-of-hours work prior to 2004.

Where does NHS 111 fit in?

NHS 111 is a free non-emergency-number medical helpline which has operated in England, Scotland (NHS 24) and Wales (NHS 111 Wales) since 2014. It replaced the nurse-led NHS Direct healthcare advice service.

The service is staffed by trained health advisors (non-clinicians) who use a triage tool called NHS Pathways to guide their decisions. NHS England issued guidance in 2015 to integrate NHS 111 and GP out-of-hours services, meaning patients in need of care would have just one number to call to access out-of-hours care, no matter their location. The service operates 24 hours a day and can redirect patients to their own surgeries in-hours; then between 6.30pm and 8am, at weekends and Bank Holidays, to an out-of-hours service. NHS 111 has been criticised for sending a high proportion of callers to A&E.[22]

To reduce inefficiency and to try to provide a patient with a complete episode of care, from 2017 an integrated urgent care clinical assessment service (IUC CAS) was introduced, making senior GPs available to callers, with the ability to prescribe electronically if needed, along with advanced nurse practitioners, paramedics, pharmacists and dental nurses.

NHS 111 played a major role in the nation's response to the Covid-19 pandemic. Many GPs came out of retirement to staff the service, and a dedicated Covid-19 clinical assessment service (CCAS) was commissioned to free up other areas of the healthcare system and help manage those most at risk of complications. In January 2023, 1.8 million calls were made to the service. This figure surged to 3 million at the start of the pandemic in March 2020.[23]

Since 2020, GP practices have been contractually required to free up appointments for direct booking by NHS 111, leading to GPs being overwhelmed with demand. The 2021 England LMC conference heard from GPs that the 111 service was 'not fit for purpose' with patients frequently being booked into GP slots for non-urgent issues.[24]

NHS commissioning and privatisation

Commissioning (the process of planning, securing and monitoring services) was introduced to the NHS in the early 1990s, when the 'internal market' was born. 'Internal' because both buyers and sellers of services were NHS organisations. Until 1989, health authorities decided which services were needed and provided it through their own hospitals. Margaret Thatcher's government introduced these market theories into health care on the belief that making providers compete for resources would encourage greater efficiency and innovation.

Entire books have been written on this topic, but in brief, since the Thatcher years, successive governments have made incremental changes to the NHS to open it up to privatisation. In secondary care, large numbers of private finance initiative (PFI) contracts outsourced NHS buildings and their maintenance to private companies, burdening the NHS with colossal debts. Tony Blair's Labour government took on huge numbers of PFI projects, in which private companies covered the upfront costs of building or maintaining hospitals, which they then owned, and then went on to lease back to the NHS. In 2020–1, hospitals spent £2.3 billion on legacy PFI projects, with close to £0.5 billion alone being spent on interest charges (equivalent to the salaries of 15,000 newly qualified nurses).[25] Some NHS trusts have been paying more on PFI repayments than they spent on medications.[26]

Back in primary care, the reforms of the 1990s saw the introduction of the fundholding scheme, which for the first time gave GPs a budget for commissioning. The Labour government scrapped this in 1997, only to reintroduce it as 'practice-based commissioning' a few years later (2005–13).

Reorganisation is a common endeavour when it comes to the NHS, and a cycle of acronyms have been assigned to these reforms – essentially renaming the organisations who work together to plan and pay for health and care services. Primary care groups (PCGs, 1999–2002) became primary care trusts (PCTs, 2002–13), which became clinical commissioning groups (CCGs, 2013–22), which became integrated care systems (ICSs, 2022–present).

Andrew Lansley's Health and Social Care Act of 2012 introduced huge sweeping reforms across the NHS, including the creation of NHS England and CCGs. For the very first time, the NHS was given operational independence from the government. NHS England became the accountable party rather than the Health Secretary. It enforced competition between the NHS, private firms and charities, making it easier for private companies to acquire NHS contracts.

Since then, we've seen vast amounts of public funds directed to the private sector. Private companies have been able to take on lucrative contracts, cherry-picking the more profitable areas, and then just pack up shop and leave if things go wrong. Babylon is an example of a private company that pioneered digital health care in 2017 with their app, GP at Hand. This app allowed patients to deregister from their own GP (removing the funding as they left) to sign up with the app with the promise of online appointments with Babylon GPs. Those signing up tended to be under the age of 40, with less complex medical needs, meaning NHS practices were left with the more complex patients and with even less funding to provide for them.[27] Babylon started winding down unprofitable NHS contracts in 2019, leaving large cohorts of patients without care, illustrating how relationships with private companies are focused on profit margins – the polar opposite to the premise of the NHS.

Fast forward to the height of the Covid-19 pandemic when over £500 million was spent on management consultants, hired to advise the government, using these consultants has been associated with inefficiency.[28]

NHS in the devolved nations

NHS England is the focus of much of this book, mainly because many of the legislative changes and contracts imposed upon GPs that have impacted the current state of the service were within NHS England. Privatisation has also infiltrated England much more.

Wales and the other devolved nations often get forgotten when the NHS is discussed in the media. The NHS in England, Wales,

Scotland and Northern Ireland are four separate entities with different leaders, systems and governance (NHS England, Wales and Scotland and Health and Social Care (Northern Ireland)). Since 1948, devolution has happened in a series of steps. For the Welsh NHS, legislation was passed in 1969 that separated NHS Wales from the English system, with governance under the Welsh Office of government. In 1999, responsibility was fully devolved to the Welsh Senedd (and in Scotland to the Scottish Parliament, in Northern Ireland to the Northern Ireland Assembly).

Devolution has allowed each nation to shape their healthcare systems to suit the priorities of their citizens. The biggest example of this is with NHS prescriptions. These are free for all patients in all three devolved nations, but they are only free in England if patients meet a list of criteria.

In Wales since 2009, seven local health boards (LHBs) have been delivering health services. These boards are both commissioners and providers of services (unlike with the English model). Scotland runs a system of integrated health boards, similar to Wales, while Northern Ireland has a single government department responsible for health and social care known as the Health Services Executive.

There are three NHS trusts in Wales, with an all-Wales remit: the Welsh Ambulance Service; the Velindre NHS Trust, which provides specialist cancer services; and Public Health Wales. Regulation is led by Healthcare Inspectorate Wales (HIW) (the equivalent of the Care Quality Commission (CQC) in England).

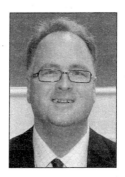

NHS GPs aren't private companies

Dr David Wrigley is a GP partner in Carnforth, Lancashire, and deputy chair of the BMA's GP Committee in England. This is adapted from a piece he wrote when the 2013 reforms had just been pushed through. The content remains relevant today.[29]

All you GPs are private providers anyway.

I often have this charge thrown at me when I speak at NHS campaign meetings. Those who level this charge at me are often those arguing in favour of a privatised NHS.

They will say that ever since 1948 GPs have been private companies, so not much is changing.

Nothing could be further from the truth.

It is true that GPs are self-employed and have been since 1948. They often own the GP surgery that they work from, and the NHS pays the GPs to allow them to employ the staff, pay for the electricity and lighting in the surgery and take home their own income too. GPs do earn a good income.

But the vast majority earn nowhere near the telephone number salaries the *Daily Mail* talk about. GPs cannot sell or advertise surgeries or set up a practice wherever they like.

And GP partners stay at their surgery through thick and thin. They invest in a community. Even during the bad times, they stay with their patients and ensure their surgery is the best it can be. We are not answerable to shareholders wishing to maximise return on their investment by increasing profit margins.

The private sector will hand the keys back and move on when the profits begin to fall; they don't want to hang around if their profit margin suffers or the shareholders start to complain.

These points are glossed over by those misleadingly claiming that GPs are an example of how NHS privatisation is nothing new.

In 2004, New Labour introduced the concept of 'alternative providers of medical services'. It allowed contracts to be held by the private sector, including by non-GPs. It gave companies like Virgin and Care UK a foothold in general practice, though hiding behind the NHS logo. It was a defining moment for general practice, and many feel the BMA GP Committee should have resisted it harder.

The false claim that 'GP practices are just businesses' was given a massive push towards reality in 2014, when it emerged that NHS England agreed, due to competition law, that *all* new GP contracts would be opened up to bids from the profit-making, private corporate sector. And – whilst struggling under funding cuts – would have to fight off the private sector to keep their practice every 5 years – signalling the rapid corporatisation of general practice.

The Health and Social Care Act of 2012 opened up the English

NHS to many more private providers. Tory and Liberal Democrat ministers repeatedly promised us that the NHS would not be forced to tender services to the private sector. Yet this is what happened to the cornerstone of the NHS, your local GP.

Competition became the name of the game and billions of our taxpayers' pounds is still being wasted on legal fees, accountancy fees, management consultancy fees and complex tendering exercises – all to satisfy the demands of the Tory-led coalition.

The modern NHS
I pick up the story to give insights into today's NHS.

Chris Ham's recent King's Fund Report[30] describes succinctly what has happened since the year 2000 within the NHS. For the first decade of the new millennium, funding increases resulted in major improvements in NHS performance. This clearly demonstrated that if the political will exists, and leaders take a longer-term perspective, then the NHS is capable of great things. Following substantial increases in staffing and pay, that decade saw a huge reduction in waiting times for most hospital treatments and greater access to GP services.[31]

In April 1999, the National Institute for Clinical Excellence (NICE) was established to deliver consistent, evidence-based guidance to the NHS on what are both clinically and cost-effective drugs and treatments. Public health measures such as the 2007 smoking ban in public places prioritised health promotion and preventative medicine, as did the launch of initiatives such as the NHS bowel screening programme (which detects an estimated 3,000 cancers each year) and the human papilloma virus (HPV) vaccination programme to prevent cervical cancer.

The Shipman Inquiry reached its conclusions in 2005, leaving a lasting impression on how general practice is regulated. GP Harold Shipman was exposed as a serial killer, responsible for the deaths of up to 215 patients. The public's faith in the medical profession was understandably shaken by this revelation following his high-profile trial. A host of regulatory changes were introduced following the inquiry, including safer management of controlled drugs and monitoring of prescribing data, systems to monitor mortality rates and unexpected deaths, changes to the death certification process and the introduction of revalidation and appraisals of GPs, alongside GP practice inspections.[32]

From 2010 onwards, NHS performance began its decline, in line with much lower funding and neglect of workforce planning. The coalition government of 2010–15 and the Conservative government that followed, imposed over a decade of austerity, opting for short-term fixes rather than longer-term solutions. As a result, we have seen stress increasing across all services, especially in mental health, learning disability services, primary care and community services.[33] Improvements in population health stalled or went into reverse after 2010 as public health failed to be prioritised or funded. Perhaps the most shocking statistic to share is that life expectancy for the most deprived people in the UK decreased over this same period.[34]

Between 2010 and 2019, the social care sector had £8 billion stripped from the adult social care budgets, according to Age UK.[35] Staff have left the sector in droves. The impact of this upon the rest of the health service is immense. Medically fit patients with social care needs are unable to leave acute hospital beds because of the lack of social care provision. This puts pressure on the rest of the system, leaving patients waiting on trolleys in corridors in emergency departments, or even further back in the queue, still inside ambulances waiting to be seen. The cost of keeping a medically fit patient in an NHS bed is three times the cost of keeping them in a nursing home.[36]

In 2020, when the Covid-19 pandemic hit, this crisis exposed the impacts of a decade of insufficient NHS funding. In early 2020, shortages of ventilators and intensive care beds were major concerns, and later in the pandemic, capacity constraints hindered attempts of staff working through backlogs in elective care.[37] In 2022, there were nearly 40,000 excess deaths (meaning more people dying than would be expected, above the 5-year average figures).[38] The pandemic itself impacted this figure of course, but the number has not yet levelled, as would be expected post-pandemic. The number for 2022 was similar to that of 2019. We know there were about 2,200 additional deaths in England in the winter 2022, and this was associated with A&E delays. Factors such as poverty, inequality and an under resourced health system have all combined with a cost-of-living crisis to cost people their lives.

The NHS has now reached retirement age and is currently in need of life support. Today, the NHS, and society as a whole, are very different to the NHS and society of 1948. The NHS has adapted over the years, but the current pressures are undeniable. Radical solutions are needed to bring the service back to life.

Chapter 2
How the role has changed

Writing about the NHS and health care can be very clinical and impersonal. Facts and figures do set the scene, but we need to hear stories from people that have experienced a changing NHS. When training to become a GP, I recall, for the first time in my many years of studying, seeing a list of suggested reading. What was unusual about the list was that not one of the books was a medical textbook; they were all tales about patients, doctors, people's lives and their stories. The power of a good story is universal.

One book that GPs are routinely encouraged to read is a book from 1967 called *A Fortunate Man*,[39, 40] which traces 6 weeks in the life of a country doctor, working in a remote valley on the Welsh/English border. Hailed as one of the most important books ever written about general practice, it follows John Sassall's evolution as a doctor, through the stories of his patients, illustrated with photos of the landscape in which they live.

In the summer of 2020, writer Polly Morland stumbled across this book when clearing out her mother's house. She recognised the photos in the book as being the valley she lived in, inspiring her to contact the valley's current doctor and tell an updated account of a rural GP, resulting in her book: *A Fortunate Woman*.[41]

Medicine has changed dramatically since 1967, and despite the fallout from the pandemic and rocketing workloads, *A Fortunate Woman* beautifully captures the reasons many of my contemporaries became GPs. It also shines a light on the importance of relationship-based care.

The stories and experiences of GPs are rarely shared, maybe due to fears of breaching patient confidentiality or worries about damaging relationships or losing trust. Indeed, the doctor in Morland's book remains anonymous.

As a patient in Morland's book says, her GP is 'a person, not a service', and that is too easily forgotten in this current world. This chapter focuses on hearing from the people behind the service, and their stories of an evolving NHS.

Thirty years as a Cornish GP

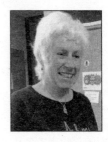

Dr Christine Hunter worked as a GP in Cornwall from 1985 to 2017. She tells me how the profession has changed throughout the span of her career.

Christine Hunter has general practice in her blood. Her father started working as a country GP in Shetland immediately after the Second World War, at the very inception of the NHS. 'My medical career started with sitting in his dispensary as a small child, helping him with prescriptions,' she said. 'I loved the way our family were a part of the community, and this was how I saw the role of a family doctor.'

Dr Hunter completed her GP training in Newquay, Cornwall, in 1985, and recalls her weekly tutorials involving a read over the local paper to catch up on important news about patients – from births, marriages and deaths, to the court pages. The world of general practice in the 1980s was a different one to that which we operate in today. The miners' strikes came to an end in 1985. This was also the year of Live Aid and the very first episode of long-running soap *EastEnders*. It was a time when pubs were still smoky and, only 2 years before, they could refuse to serve women based on gender alone. Computers were not in widespread use (although the first GP to use a computer in his consulting room was a Dr John Preece from Exeter in 1970[42]) and mobile phones had just been invented. GPs relied on landlines, while many patients made use of public telephone boxes. It was not uncommon for a doctor to return home from a night visit to find a message waiting with the address of another patient who needed a visit.

After qualifying, Dr Hunter went on to locum in another practice in Newquay, eventually becoming a partner there in March 1987. She was pregnant with her first baby and took maternity leave within a few months:

> *My original training practice told me bluntly that although they liked me and had no complaints about my work, they didn't want a young female partner, as I would inevitably go off on maternity leave. They appointed a male trainee as a partner instead. It was definitely harder for a woman to get into partnership then for that*

reason. The practice got 13 weeks of payment to cover maternity leave which was equivalent to about 75 per cent of cost of locum cover. Some practices deducted the difference from your drawings, but that didn't happen in mine. After the 3 months, you had to pay the locum yourself if you wanted more time off, which I couldn't have afforded. It also meant I didn't get any leave allowance for the rest of the year as it was considered I had used that up in my 13 weeks of maternity leave.

She was back at work (including night visits and weekends) when her baby girl was 9 weeks old and still breastfeeding. As the children grew, she recalls 24 hours on calls, and juggling childcare with the job, which occasionally involved taking a toddler to the undertakers to complete cremation paperwork.

I really think he had no idea what was happening but did tell his grandma he'd been with mummy to a lady in bed. The children used to come with me on Christmas Day to the local cottage hospital to see the patients. They would be taken round the beds and sometimes were given a chocolate.

Night duty was generally done from home with all calls redirected to our home phone. If I had to go out on a call, my husband had to take calls and look after our baby, meaning he was tied to being at home whenever I was out. A lot of male doctors paid their wives to do this role and claimed against tax, but this didn't work out if the spouse already had a job.

I felt some resentment as I had to pay childcare to be able to work and any extra hours I had to do would cost me. Male GPs didn't have this to worry about and expected me to be available at short notice to fill in for them on holidays. Since I was only part time, it was assumed I had the flexibility to fill their days off and wouldn't get any more money.

Things started to change in the 1990s when a local GP cooperative started, complete with a call handler, booked clinics and cars with equipment and a driver. My last ever night shift I did was the night Princess Diana died in 1997.

I've lived in the practice area throughout my career. My children attended local schools, and I have always taken an interest in local

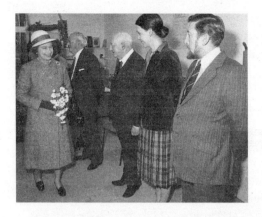

Dr Hunter's father met the Queen, when she visited The Shetland Islands in 1981

activities. I regularly meet patients out and about and always say hello and chat if stopped and this to me has always been an important part of being a family doctor.

This ethos was undoubtedly cultivated through her childhood in Shetland, where she recalls many memories of watching her father work. 'The surgery, dispensary and waiting room were a part of our house,' she explains.

He did 2 hours of surgery every day, all without appointments so anyone could turn up, with anything. I opened the door one Sunday afternoon to a gentleman who had been trout fishing in a nearby loch and had a fishhook in his eyebrow. In those days the telephone was the main way to contact. As children we weren't allowed to touch the phone as it was vital for his work. When a bit older I was allowed to take the calls in the morning when folk would ring through their prescriptions. It was usually a list of 'a box of blue tablets, a box of the little white ones and some of the white mixture'. My dad would visit an area of the island each day and people would know his schedule and request a call that day. It was mostly just a social round and a chat and very occasionally a 'wee dram'. I remember occasionally an emergency call when my mum would have to ring round to find him and redirect him.

One year the snow in the village was so bad he couldn't get the car up the hill outside the house and a girl went into labour about a mile away. Her husband walked down to meet my dad, and as he was not so fit, the young man carried him part way up the hill to see to his wife. I believe she was taken out in a helicopter in the end which was very unusual in the 1970s.

Her father retired in 1978, leaving his daughter some of his medical equipment, pictured here.

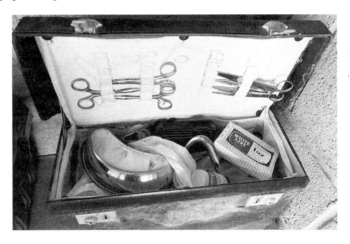

Dr Hunter became a senior partner in 2004, and retired in 2017, almost 30 years to the day since she joined. 'I have to confess, I was burnt out by then and just needed a bit of time to myself,' she said. She adds:

I had returned to locum work in my old practice by summer 2017, so I didn't really take that time, and I still do around 40 days a year of locum work even now.

Yesterday in clinic I started thinking of all the changes I've seen in general practice over the years. Most are due to improving health care and better use of doctors' time (or basic lack of it) but some do illustrate the change in the model of a family doctor from cradle to grave. Social visits to the elderly used to be a regular occurrence. My partner used to go once a week to a lady with arthritis and check her food cupboards, opening tins and jars for her meals throughout the week. We used to do antenatal clinics with the midwife, bereavement visits to the family and post-natal visits in the first week. None of this is practical now.

The magic
of general practice

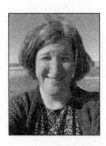

Dr Louise Hyde is a GP in Borth, Wales.

GP practices work like a small business. They are contracted out to the NHS and run by GP partners. Most GP partners are not trained in business; their main interest is in providing clinical care to patients. Over the last 10 years, there have been multiple changes to the General Medical Services (GMS) contract and how it is funded, and to survive, practices have adapted. We are now at the point where the GMS contract cannot be delivered for the money that is attached to it. Over the years, we have compensated for this by taking on extra work that makes a slight profit: running a dispensary, putting in contraceptive implants, treating minor injuries, looking after our local cottage hospital, carrying out palliative care in the community and treating our diabetic patients to an expert level in the surgery. These are all extra bits of work we do to keep the core GMS service of seeing patients who want to be seen running.

Seeing patients who want to be seen is a more complicated job than our politicians realise. When it is done well, by a GP with enough time and skill, who knows the patient, their family, the community and the context through which that patient's illness presents then this is what I call the 'magic' of general practice. This is the element of the work that can be the most satisfying for doctors, and the most valuable for patients. This is the reason why GP partners are working harder and harder doing extra jobs. It is so that they can continue to fund their core job and do it well. This is the bit that is hardest to measure and quantify, and the easiest to undervalue and underfund.

When there were enough doctors around who wanted to become permanent GP partners in our little businesses, this way of working extra jobs to fund our main job to keep it magical wasn't such a problem. But over the last 10 years, life in the UK has become harder and harder for our junior doctors doing their GP or consultant training, so those who can, have gone abroad to train.

Now we have a national GP recruitment crisis, and we need to attract the GPs back, but under current conditions we can't.

A far greater proportion of those GPs we train in the UK than ever before are becoming locums. There is plenty of work for them, so job security is not an issue. They can name their terms and their price, work when they want to and take time off when they like. As a group, their income is growing, in line with the market for their skills.

In contrast, GP partners take responsibility for providing a service to a specific group of patients (a 7,000-patient practice is about average), for funding that doesn't match up and is ever decreasing, while our workload is growing in ways that are hard to control or even quantify. Is it any wonder we are having trouble persuading locum GPs to join us as partners? They have never fully experienced the magic of general practice to the extent we have, when it encompasses the deep knowledge of our patients and their community. Even if they had, would it be attractive enough to compensate for the overworking and lack of control they would have of their lives? We need to attract these locums into permanent GP practice, but we can't.

The pandemic has added a new dimension to this problem. Not only is everyone run down, sicker and more likely to need medical care, we changed the way we arranged access to our GPs overnight.

In the early days of the Covid-19 pandemic, this change in access was purely for infection control; to minimise the number of sick people in our waiting rooms potentially spreading disease. Telephone triage and telephone consultations became the norm, and we were able to minimise how many patients we saw face to face, saving that method of contact for those where an examination would change the clinical outcome.

This change had two big side-effects. First, it diluted the magic. It's much harder to connect with someone when you can't see them; you can't use your body language, and everything has to be done through tone of voice. It's harder to make someone feel heard, and it's harder to know exactly how they are feeling or what they are thinking. It's easier to miss the clues and cues that help you interpret what they say and what they don't say, and to fill in the context of how their body moves and exists in the world. This is why we've suffered a kick-back from the general public, fuelled by right-wing media, for continuing to use telephone triage and telephone consulting as a tool.

The second side-effect is less obvious to the public, but it is the one that has made telephone triage very hard to give up. Suddenly, we can see the overview, and the full extent of the need that's out there in our communities. It's overwhelming.

With growing poverty, a pandemic that's ongoing but largely ignored, and a social infrastructure suffering from years of underfunding and neglect, our population is sicker than ever before. Triage allows us to prioritise, to delegate, signpost or reroute, and to use our time as efficiently as possible to meet the enormous needs of our communities. This method is not popular. Part of the magic of a GP is that they will always be there, always accessible in times of need. They are known, if not personally, then at least by reputation.

Other clinicians can do finite bits of what a GP does. Pharmacists, physiotherapists and nurse practitioners can take on well-defined areas of work very safely and competently now that GPs have to save time to do the work that only a GP can do. The continuity that patients and GPs values highly, and that we know saves lives, is further eroded.

We are moving mountains of workload in general practice now, doing our level best to provide a service that is as safe and efficient as possible, given the huge new demands. But that comes at a cost; there is a risk of losing the magic.

I still love my job, but I don't want to spend every waking moment of my life doing it. I want to preserve as much of the magic as possible, and I want to share the magic of general practice with my colleagues. And I want more of those colleagues to share it with.

If you value the magic of general practice, too, please ask your assembly member or MP to start adequately funding our core GMS services to match the increased needs of our population, because that is where the magic is.

Save our surgeries – NHS Wales

GPs in Wales have urged the Welsh government to produce a workforce strategy to save general practice. The BMA reported a deficit of 664 GPs in Wales in 2023,[43] following the closure of 84 surgeries in the last 10 years. Those practices that remain open are absorbing the work, with the average list size in Wales increasing from 6,780 to 8,378.

Workload continues to rise, and in 2022–3, GPs in Wales took 27 million telephone contacts, offered 19 million appointments, issued 56 million (free!) prescription items, along with over 500,000 sick notes, and made 1.3 million referrals to secondary care.

The campaign asks for restored funding for general practice in Wales, alongside investment in the workforce, to ensure enough GPs are trained and retained, with a focus on improving staff wellbeing.

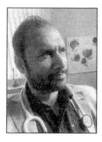

Expert generalism – the power, the magic and the pitfalls

Dr Ayan Panja is a GP partner in St Albans. He is a lifestyle medicine educator, author, podcaster, former BBC World News presenter and editorial advisor to NHS Digital.

General practice is dying. The days of consulting with a doctor who knows you – really knows you – are rapidly vanishing.

Some modernists would argue that this doesn't matter, and that knowing your doctor is a sentimental luxury. In the modern world of artificial intelligence (AI) and accurate diagnostics, it's the diagnosis that matters, right? Who cares whether it's by a machine or a person? And surely a machine is more accurate. Perhaps this part of the process is true for rare conditions, and as much as I love technology as a powerful adjunct to consulting a doctor, the true strength of general practice has been continuity and the expert generalist skillset.

Firstly, someone needs to have a broad overview of the issue and be able to diagnose, explain, support and contextualise. These, and the power of prediction, are the superpowers of a generalist. Professor Philip Tetlock often talks about how generalists are better at predicting outcomes when compared to specialists.[44] There has, however, been an increasing trend towards specialisation. The world seems to value specialist opinion, and this is mirrored in science and technology, with sub-specialities in most disciplines. Medicine is no exception, where an eye surgeon now no longer deals with the whole eye: one surgeon deals with the eyelid;

another with the retina; someone else, glaucoma; and another with the cataracts. This world is a different one to the one we had 30 years ago.

In primary care, where resources are scarce, the hidden generalist values in a GP being able to contextualise a patient's symptoms quickly, having known you and your back story for years, is only one part of GP 'magic'. Other skills include being able to amass and filter an enormous amount of information, coordinating and analysing results and correspondence, whilst dealing with several other issues in the same consultation. This often happens effortlessly, meaning that it can pass as unseen work, as the GP is effectively constantly 'sweeping up'.

With fragmented episodic care, which is what we are seeing more of, all of the work mentioned above can bounce around. The system then becomes more expensive and inefficient, with more work duplication and patients feeling uncared for. The lack of a full sweep up of issues means another contact is often needed with a different practitioner. This in itself can lead to a sense of dissatisfaction as a patient. 'Who is actually in charge of my care here?' is not an uncommon thought.

The GP has historically been a continuous sweeper for allcomers when it comes to a patient's problems, whereas fragmented care is just as it sounds – incomplete. A lot gets left behind, and guess who has to deal with that. It all comes back to the GP anyway, a member of a workforce that is diminishing day by day.

Add into all this the fact that much of the work GPs see does not fit into guidelines; generalist skills are essential to hone things down. The GP is like a good detective. 'I feel shaky on the inside quite a lot…' isn't a description you will find in the textbooks, but it is one that may make more sense to a doctor and patient who have known each other for years. There are also curses to being a trusted generalist. GPs are human and make mistakes, increasingly so as the workload and pressure ramp up. And as we are often closer to our patients than our colleagues in hospitals, their frustrations are often taken out on us. This is a little bit like people sharing their stresses with their family members, except via a letter of complaint. But we continue to do our best.

Even if you are convinced by this argument for generalism and continuity, the sad reality is that there are not enough GPs for the people who need our services: people are sicker, there is more need, and more work gets dumped on the waning GP service. The workload is becoming unsustainable, and we are burning out rapidly.

What does the solution look like? Some talk about a segmentation of patients where those who need continuity get it: people with complex needs, the elderly and the vulnerable. A cast of clinical characters support GPs and take some of the load: our incredibly steadfast nursing colleagues, paramedics, pharmacists and physiotherapists all support us whilst we still maintain that overview.

There is also value in groups. The increasing lack of true community these days means that there is now a real case for creating them via shared health needs. Health coaches are perfectly placed to do this, and every GP surgery is now able to bring them on board. Something powerful happens in groups that doesn't happen in one-to-one situations (think parkrun or Weight Watchers). People's greatest asset is other people and group medicine is still in its infancy in the UK. And for those who love the long-term relationship built on trust with their own doctor, group medicine is perfect and moves people away from statements such as: 'Only Dr X understands…I need to speak to her…' But group medicine alone is not enough. We need more investment in primary care, a system that used to work beautifully most of the time and is now broken. We cannot expect people to tolerate a service that is this stretched or expect GPs to be able to work within it as it stands.

We remain at the mercy of the state and it's high time for GPs and patients to voice their concerns together.

Chapter 3
GPs and the pandemic

The pandemic caused a seismic shift in how GP practices function. As Covid hit our shores in March 2020, NHS England mandated the move to 'total triage' in primary care to limit the spread of the virus to protect both patients and staff.[45] Almost overnight, GPs shifted to remote telephone, video and online consults. 'Hot hubs' were established to enable ongoing face-to-face contact if the clinical need arose. Contrary to what became the propaganda of the pandemic 'Your GP surgery is closed', GP teams were barely pausing for breath. Days off were forfeited as we had to try to make sense of ever-changing guidelines and Covid restrictions, while also trying to define the 'new normal'. Supplies of PPE were sorely lacking in primary care[46] and as a consequence, many GPs were among those healthcare workers who lost their lives.[47]

As the pandemic endured, GP teams delivered, at short notice, 75 per cent of a mass new vaccination programme,[48] while simultaneously juggling the backlogs resulting from cancelled secondary care work. Data from NHS digital[49] confirmed that, contrary to the reports of being closed, general practice was busier than ever before, with over a million more appointments being offered in September 2020 compared to 2019.[50] Not only were GPs busier, but the work was also more complex, since remote consults are inherently riskier from a medicolegal perspective. They also often take longer than a face-to-face review.

Undoubtedly, there were, and still are, problems accessing care. A report by the patients watchdog Healthwatch asked over 200,000 people about their experiences of accessing GPs during the pandemic.[51] The group found that while remote appointments were more convenient for many, they weren't for everyone, leaving some patients worried that their health problems 'will not be accurately diagnosed'. The report found that some patients struggled to get appointments for more routine health check-ups. Issues with the communication of these changes was the main take-home message, with Healthwatch saying that GPs must prioritise telling patients that they are open for face-to-face appointments.

Statements like this illustrate the power of the media. GPs were open, but there was a strong press narrative that practices were closed to patients and that GPs were hiding away. So powerful was the message, drip fed over months, that GPs were being asked 'When are you re-opening?' by patients sitting in front of them mid consult in an open GP surgery. This degree of disconnect is almost impossible to counter. The constant trickle of GP negativity from some sections of the media, coupled with difficulty navigating new ways of working, left many patients, and sadly many secondary care colleagues, upset and angry about their (incorrect) belief that GPs had closed down and did not work throughout the pandemic.

The Spectator	**Daily Mail**
It's time for NHS GPs to stop hiding behind their telephones	**LET'S GET BACK TO SEEING GPs FACE TO FACE**

More worrying were those people that stayed away due to this messaging: the person with a breast lump; people with chronic conditions they let lapse to avoid 'bothering anyone' or the lady with a heart attack, who sat at home for weeks with chest pain because 'you were closed'. The consequences of these false narratives are deadly serious.

'There is mounting anger that a highly rewarded and once highly respected profession continues to insist that it is "fully open" when personal experience suggests it is hiding behind an increasingly threadbare Covid sofa,' began one commentator in the *Telegraph*.[52] 'Who is backing those GPs who don't want to return to normal working because – unlike shopworkers, waiters, district nurses and delivery drivers – they are at risk from a fast receding virus?'

The reason you can't see your GP, is not because of their laziness or

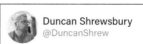

Duncan Shrewsbury
@DuncanShrew

GP is, and has been throughout, OPEN.
Pat exp is variable, we know & bits we could do better - we are trying (& sorry).
But when you have a patient *in* a F2F appt asking when you're opening again, it begs the question what messages are circulating & how they're understood

lack of engagement. The data tells the story of just how hard the workforce has been toiling. You can't see your GP because the workforce has been in decline since 2015. Funding has been static and GPs are paid around £163.65 per patient per year (this is similar to the cost of one private GP consult, and half the cost of one hospital outpatient appointment). When demand goes up, this funding doesn't increase. GPs are just asked to work harder. And GPs and their teams *have* worked harder. Working 12–14 hours a day, while being branded lazy, is a bitter pill to swallow.

Sara Macbay
@Saramac7

Replying to @HelenRSalisbury @DAUK_GP and 14 others

I had 25 pt contacts booked for this afternoon alone, having done my 44 bed care home ward round in the morning & all the jobs that generates. I got home at 10pm. We are given 5 mins for tel triage. Simply not possible. Will log in on day off tom to do admin unpaid.

Lizzi Helsby
@Lizzimooneydoc

Replying to @DAUK_GP

This morning I had 28 tel calls, 8 f2f. 56 prescriptions, 30 documents to read. 2 calls from ambulance crew and a home visit. Then the afternoon starts .... 😔 oh yeah and 3 letters from consultants asking me to order tests and bloods because they did a tel call to the pt

I'm a GP & seen patients daily F2F: @ surgery, @ home visit, care homes, hospital wards, A&E depts, police custody, prison, in street, a tent, their car. In hours + night & weekend. On phone, on video, in person. When a few days old & when dying Yet @NHSEngland implies we're shut

It was even more demoralising when NHS England decided to throw GPs under the bus. Instead of quashing the well-documented negativity from the press,[53] our leaders perpetuated this narrative, with a press release in September 2020 reminding GPs to offer face-to-face appointments, which fuelled further angry headlines.[54] Deflated GPs then faced increasing complaints and abuse from patients, culminating in one practice being daubed in graffiti[55] and another subject to an arson attack[56] (see 'Rising levels of abuse towards GPs' by Dr Aman Amir). Primary care medical director, Dr Nikki Kanani, later apologised on X (formerly Twitter) for the 'conclusions drawn by the media'.[57] Little had changed a year later, with violence escalating and four practice staff being hospitalised.[58] In Wales, Michele Richards, a practice manager at a surgery in Newport, called the police twice in one week to report aggressive patients.[59] A receptionist had been punched, while another had been racially abused. 'The abuse we are facing is horrific,' she told WalesOnline, 'GPs have put themselves at risk throughout the pandemic and we're working harder than ever. The idea that we've been shut and aren't doing anything is just soul destroying.'

The pandemic has affected every part of the health service. Secondary care was required to make similar adaptations, cancelling routine work and moving to telephone clinics without facing the same vitriol that primary care suffered. 'People waiting months, if not years for hospital outpatient appointments and elective surgery are turning to GPs for medication, updates and extra help. People who have minor problems that they delayed getting attention for last year are finding that the problems are no longer minor,' said Michele. 'When patients do get through to us they're absolutely frustrated because it's taken them so long. By the time they speak to us all the appointments for the day have already been allocated. It's not a case of us being lazy, it's just that demand is outstripping capacity.'

Ultimately, the ones who suffer the most in this game of political point scoring are the patients. But instead of being angry at those in power for their lack of GP appointments, the messaging has been cleverly weaved so the GPs have become the bad guys.

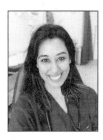

Being a GP during the pandemic

Dr Neena Jha is a GP in Hertfordshire.

I remember the start of the pandemic so vividly, yet the rest feels like a blur: the call to action, the adrenaline kick and the hunger for knowledge – almost an obsession, about how the virus was spreading around the world, getting closer and wondering if and when it would reach us. When Covid finally hit our shores, it felt like everything changed overnight.

There was a national shift in attitude that I had never experienced before: an astounding feeling of determination and togetherness, initially, anyway.

As a healthcare professional, it was quite overwhelming. It felt like the weight of responsibility had been placed squarely on our shoulders and we had no choice but to live up to the nation's expectations of being 'the heroes'. I distinctively remember hearing healthcare staff described as 'soldiers going to war', putting their lives on the line to protect the country. And that's exactly how it felt. What brought that aspect home for me was seeing our senior GP partner who is in his early sixties, who'd had a thick moustache for almost his entire adult life, turn up to work clean shaven. I stopped in my tracks and felt a wave of emotion. He feared his facial hair would impact the tight seal of his face mask which could be a safety hazard. It felt like a wakeup call that shifted from a theoretical risk to our lives due to our job role to a very real one. I remember seeing the news when the first NHS worker died of Covid, then the second, the third and all too quickly it became too many to count.

The workload seemed never-ending. Covid guidelines were changing constantly; just keeping yourself updated felt like a full-time job. Access changed overnight. In primary care, as well as in most hospital outpatient clinics, consultations were changed from face to face to an initial telephone triage approach, as directed by NHS England to reduce the rate of viral transmission. We implemented community Covid hot sites where we could separate our Covid and non-Covid patients. There were significant and rapidly evolving changes to access that patients and staff had to adjust to.

Something I certainly had not expected was the change in public perception towards healthcare staff, particularly those of us who worked in primary care. The 'battle against Covid' was perceived as being fought only by those staff who worked in hospital, and we saw many media outlets branding GPs as 'lazy, cowardly and closed during the pandemic'.

This could not have been further from the truth, but unfortunately these false headlines had significant consequences. For patients, who believed these headlines and did not seek medical attention, and also for staff, who experienced a notable rise in abuse. One in three GPs was a victim of either physical or verbal abuse from a patient or relative. It was shocking and incredibly upsetting to see images of foul graffiti being smeared across a GP surgery, colleagues posting on social media about threatening notes that had been sent to their surgery and most horrifically an appalling attack on a GP practice resulting in four staff members being hospitalised with injuries. The abuse, coupled with the insurmountable and often unsafe workloads, has taken an understandable toll with GPs leaving the profession at an unprecedented rate.

> **PulseToday** ☑
> @pulsetoday
>
> A man, 59, has been charged with assault after an attack on a Manchester GP practice on Friday. @gmpolice confirmed that four members of staff were injured in the incident. Two of the victims were hospitalised with head injuries

I remember making a round of tea at my practice, looking at the list on the board which had staff members' drink preferences, and seeing almost one third of the names crossed off the list. It was a visual snapshot of the crippling effects of the pandemic on the GP workforce. The staffing crisis did not affect primary care alone, as I witnessed in my other job roles.

As well as working as a GP, I undertook a few additional roles during the pandemic including working in our local hospital emergency department, the urgent care centre, 111 Herts urgent care service, the Covid vaccinator sites and the prevention of admission team.

It was definitely an eye-opener working for the NHS in different capacities, as I was able to witness pressures on different healthcare systems and how they feed into each other, particularly whilst working in the emergency department. What took me by surprise was the huge degree of overlap between primary and secondary care. I saw many 'primary care' patients, some of whom had struggled to get a face-to-face GP appointment, others who attended out of desperation at their wait times for outpatient investigations or clinic appointments. Conversely, in general practice I increasingly saw 'secondary care' patients, those who had serious and/or emergency medical issues but booked GP appointments as they struggled to endure waiting hours in A&E to be seen. It seemed that patients were understandably just accessing medical help wherever they could.

I am unsure and apprehensive of what the future holds for our NHS. It has certainly been under more strain than I have ever witnessed before. The cracks are growing ever larger, to the point where I fear they may be beyond repair. What I have seen in this pandemic is that the NHS has an abundance of dedicated, passionate and incredible staff. As a country, we would be wise to recognise and value that before it is too late.

Rising levels of abuse towards GPs

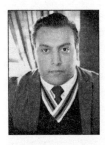

Dr Aman Amir is a GP partner in Liverpool, an author of many novels and a university lecturer and magistrate in Manchester.

I decided to become a GP in 2008. I was selected onto a 3-year general practice training programme in the northwest, rotating through various specialties including psychiatry; obstetrics and gynaecology; ear, nose and throat; infectious diseases; and of course, general practice. Like all GPs in the UK, I had to clear the membership exams to obtain my certificate of completion of training and be recognised as a fully qualified GP. The learning journey continues even now, and much time and effort must be devoted towards CPD and regular appraisals to ensure high professional standards. Like many, I had to juggle personal and professional commitments while bearing the financial and emotional expense of the training.

Since qualifying, I have worked in primary care in the northwest, holding various positions of responsibility including clinical director, lecturer and GP partner. I've supported the training and development of medical students, nursing students and physician associates along with junior doctors and GP trainees. While working as a doctor in the NHS for over 20 years, I have observed many things and tried to reflect on some of my own experiences.

My father lost his life to cancer in 1996. My mother lost hers in 2022, also to cancer. In both cases it was the GP who had the holistic approach towards their care and battled to coordinate the services to aid our family through the most difficult of times.

GPs are dealing with an ageing population with complex medical and social needs within an overstretched service with both funding and staffing issues. Appointment times are short, to offer as many as possible, yet it's very difficult to do so much in the allocated time, which is why many surgeries run late. A day's work for a GP is, of course, not just the screen of appointments. It includes the daily communications from hospitals, the medication requests, letters and home visits, unexpected emergencies, along with teaching and supervision of colleagues. It is fair to say that primary care physicians have never worked so hard. Yet it is also fair to say that we have never been so undervalued.

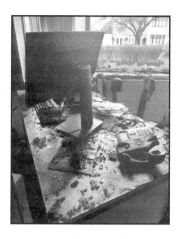 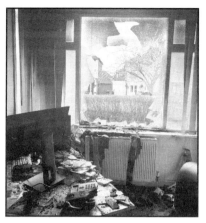

During the pandemic, we witnessed GP teams deliver successful vaccination campaigns while still providing care to communities. We cheered and clapped for the NHS. Imagine my shock and heartbreak when our practice was subjected to an arson attack in February 2022. In the early hours of that particular morning, I was informed that the surgery had been set on fire.

Windows had been smashed, and equipment charred and ruined. Luckily, no-one was hurt. The incident was widely reported, with Pulse noting that 'just days before the arson attack, racist graffiti was sprayed on the front and side of the practice with the words "paki" and "paedo" scrawled on the white walls.'

The destruction wasn't just limited to buildings and equipment. Six months later, we are still not back in the premises. The police investigations are ongoing, with no details released on who did this or why. This has had far-reaching consequences for both staff and patients. Staff are trying to work from various temporary locations and cover for those off sick. We have been unable to deliver the service we would like to, and our patients have been severely inconvenienced by delayed appointments, scripts and travel problems. The emotional and financial strain that this has caused has taken its toll on the team. Managing patient and staff expectations is already a challenging task in the NHS. The whole situation undermined the confidence the community had in their surgery.

On a personal note, this happened while I was still caring for my mother during her terminal illness. I managed to care for her and

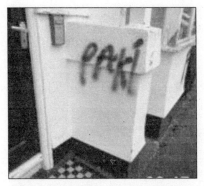

Racial slur on our surgery wall – our kind neigbour covered two. This is at Roby Medical Centre

continue to care for my patients. It was a very tricky balance and I'm proud I stuck with both.

As time passes, sympathy from patients slowly wears off and frustration seeps in, which unfortunately adds to the cycle of discontentment. My concern is that this might add to the potential abuse general practice gets, moving forward.

We continue to work very hard to try to deliver high standards of care at a difficult time. We value the need to train and develop the doctors and nurses of the future and see the time spent on this as good investment for the future of our communities. We need to nurture an environment that respects and values our healthcare teams and supports them so that they can help and support communities in their times of need.

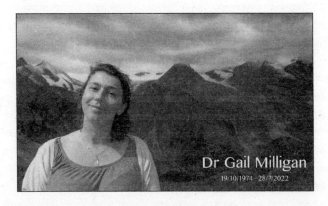

Dr Gail Milligan
19/10/1974 - 28/7/2022

The personal toll of being a GP

Dr Gail Milligan, a GP in Surrey, took her own life in July 2022 after the pressures of her job became too much to bear. Her husband, Chris Milligan, spoke to me after he wrote the tribute below, which was widely shared on social media. He wants lessons to be learnt from what happened to Gail, for people to realise how hard GPs have been working and the impact negative public opinion has. 'I don't want anyone else to have to go through this,' he told GPonline. 'I understand people being frustrated because they can't get a doctor's appointment, but they need to know the real story of what's going on behind the scenes – that doctors are dying to offer services that they know aren't up to scratch anymore.'[60]

Gail knew she wanted to be a GP from the age of six. She graduated from Manchester University in 1998 and went on to train as a GP in Reading, becoming a partner and GP trainer at Camberley Health Centre in Surrey in 2003. She met Chris when she was 18. They married 8 years later and had two sons. 'Gail was always the one who went above and beyond,' Chris said. 'If anybody needed help, her door was always open.'

It was at the start of the pandemic, when Gail was set up with a laptop to work from home, that her workload began to spiral out of control. She was an eight-session partner with a Thursday off, but it became normal for her to work 12 to 14 hours a day, including working from home on her days off, putting in 70 to 80 hours a week – sometimes more. She lost the ability to switch off from work when she got home.

Combined with the immense workload pressures, the negative media coverage of general practice also took a toll, and Gail struggled with the claims that GPs were 'lazy' and not seeing patients face to face. Chris says that his wife experienced increased levels of abuse from patients and had people screaming at her. 'People were saying GPs were lazy,' Chris said. 'She was working herself to death.'

In a moving social media post, Chris wrote:

My wife died on Wednesday. She went missing for nearly 24 hours before a search and rescue dog team found her body in a forest. The unbearable pressure of her job finally got to her. For years she has been giving everything she had to other people in her professional life and her private life too. She really was the best of us. Her job as a partner at a GP surgery became overwhelming. Especially during the pandemic. She was seeing patients face-to-face the whole time, as well as the unbelievable amount of telephone consultations that were happening. She saw old people dying in care homes during the pandemic, and was working at the vaccine centres. She was responsible for the training of multiple GPs over the years, she was currently training three of them. She also worked with other medical organisations like the CCG and many others. All that, and patients too. The pressure of not making mistakes, and the endless emails and paperwork meant that for the last few years of her life she'd been neglecting herself. She used to leave for work at 06:45 and not get home until 19:30–20:00. When she arrived home she would generally work until I made her go to bed at 11pm. That was a 'lazy' four days a week. On her 'lazy' day off on Thursdays, she would work for about 12 hours. Meetings on Zoom and Microsoft Teams, never ending emails and calls. This tipped over into the weekends more recently. The same workload all weekend. Very recently she hasn't even had time for an hour's dog walk. All that and running the business of the practice too. Human Resources was her responsibility, and sadly, it turned out to be the thing that broke her.

Last Sunday afternoon, she opened an email that hit her so hard that she never recovered. She went into a deep, deep depression from the Monday to the Wednesday, when she took her life. We tried to intervene. Her colleagues tried as hard as they could to get her out of it. Offering to take over for her, and trying to reassure her that her thinking about a situation was wrong. And it was wrong. She had lost the ability to think rationally. Something had gone wrong in her head. By the time we realised what was happening, it was already too late. Her colleagues told her to take some time off on Wednesday afternoon, and to go home. She never came home. And never will now. Instead she drove into a forest, walked deep into it where she would be nearly impossible to find, and took her own life in the most shockingly violent way. This was not a cry for help. This was clearly the only way she could see her suffering stopping. It's been suggested that she suffered a psychotic episode. If you knew my wife, you'd know how far from normal any of this was for her. She was so proud of our boys, and would have never dreamed of doing anything to hurt them. However, mental illness had other ideas. Looking back, and talking to friends and family, I think she had been hiding it for years, while helping other people deal with their mental health, she neglected her own. It's such a sad waste of a wonderful, beautiful, funny and absolutely bananas wife, mother and doctor. All over something that had no relation to reality. The next time you hear someone banging on about lazy doctors, please stop and think about *what happened to my wife. We are in no doubt that the job made her ill. Me and my boys are broken. Especially me, I don't think I'll ever be the same again. We'd been together for thirty years this year. It was almost always lots of laughter and fun with huge amounts of piss-taking. My boys have lost their mother, and I have lost my best friend. Sorry about this post. I would like to say that normal service will resume, but it won't. I'm broken. And finally...An hour after I found out Gail was dead, I had to take our dog to be put to sleep. Aggressive cancer had torn through her at a terrific rate. She spent her last 24 hours cuddled up between two police officers on our sofa. The police stayed with me from the time I reported my wife missing until the time they found her...And a bit longer too. I will be forever grateful to Thames Valley police, and the team at Berkshire Lowland Search and Rescue, who were the team who found her. No wife. No mother to our boys. No dog. And I thought losing my dad a year ago was bad. What was I thinking? There just aren't enough GPs to cope, and now there is one less.*

NHS Practitioner Health is a primary care mental health service created to treat health and care professionals. The service logs deaths of health professionals where suicide is deemed the cause. From October 2021 to October 2022 they were aware of 18 such deaths. This number is likely to be an underestimate.[61]

Chris Milligan has voiced his concerns that general practice is no longer a safe place to work, especially for partners, and he requests that lessons are learnt from his wife's death. He advocates for workload limits for doctors; protected time for them to reflect on difficult cases and proactive intervention to support GPs who may be struggling.

Practitioner Health conducted a survey of almost 6,000 health professionals who registered as new patients with their service in the 12 months preceding October 2022. Out of those who took part, 1,836 people reported having suicidal thoughts on several days, more than half of the days or nearly every day in the 2 weeks prior to presenting for help. Of these people, just under a third (496 people) had made plans to end their lives in the last week. This figure rose by 8 per cent between 2021 and 2022. Workload pressures are now commonly cited as a reason for these suicidal thoughts, with many reporting that the demands of the job have become overwhelming and unmanageable.[62]

'I don't want this to happen to another family,' Chris said. 'I really want people to be kind to themselves and kind to each other, and not to work so bloody hard. And don't take on too many responsibilities – because that's when it can become too much and they lose themselves.'

For mental health and wellbeing resources for doctors and health professionals facing difficulties: see Help for GPs on page 154.

GPs are not lazy, we're working harder than ever

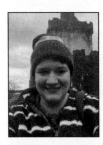

Dr Elizabeth Croton is a GP based in Birmingham. She's also a sessional doctor with NHS Practitioner Health. She's held various roles as a GP, writer and member of the DAUK's GP Committee. She wrote this piece, giving a snapshot into a typical day's work during the pandemic, for metro.co.uk in September 2021, which is reproduced here with permission.[63]

It's 8am and I'm already sat in front of my computer at the surgery. I prescribe myself some coffee and scroll through the blood results and hospital letters that have accumulated since yesterday. There are at least 100 in total. I get through as many as I can before morning surgery starts at 8.30am. I have a minimum of 32 patient contacts a day, of which a third to a half are seen in person, depending on the nature of their issue. Abdominal pains and earaches are easier to see in person, while a pill request can often be dealt with over the phone. A typical day may take me from migraine headaches and a sofa allergy to a new diagnosis of cancer.

Working as a GP has always been both an art and a science to me, and at the moment it's tougher than ever before – for both the patients struggling to adapt to a new way of interacting with their doctor and for clinicians dealing with the backlogs caused by Covid.

I've been saddened by a deluge of negative press articles[64] recently about the service that GPs provide. I hugely resent the idea that I am lazy, work-shy and doing my best to wriggle out of seeing patients when, in reality, I've never worked harder. Like most GPs, I regularly pull

11- or 12-hour days. I find that the problems my patients bring to me are taking far longer than the allocated 12 minutes to address. It takes energy to listen closely to what a patient is saying so that they feel heard. It takes skill to meld the clinical guidelines we have to the personality of the patient to come up with a management plan that makes sense. It's also incredibly rewarding, and I'd be hard-pressed to find something else I'd rather do, but helping others can take an emotional toll.

I can understand peoples' frustrations about remote consultations. As a clinician, I also find them difficult at times. I can often work a lot faster and more effectively if I have the person in front of me. However, it's not that simple in an ongoing pandemic. Many of the Covid cases I have seen recently have had relatively mild symptoms. It would be very easy to bring them in to sit in a waiting room with a vulnerable patient (and we can't have that). Some of our patients welcome virtual consults. I was talking to a lady today who loves the fact she doesn't have to drag the kids in with her and entertain them in the waiting room. They will never be appropriate for everyone, and we need a balance.

With something as complex as the NHS, it's unhelpful to scapegoat professions such as GPs, blaming them for reorganising their services to provide care in unprecedented times. We are all likely to be patients at some point and going forward I would like to see all parties working together to craft a service that meets the needs of the population it serves. In recent months, DAUK has met with patient charity HealthWatch, to gain an understanding of the difficulties patients face accessing GP services. They've called for an investigation into the problem from NHS England – which I think is a positive step.

Personally, I'd like to see the flexibility of longer appointments for patients who need more time. I'd also like to see more investment in the service to allow greater continuity of care for patients with the same GP. I struggle daily with a hollow feeling of not having the resources to do my job properly, particularly in the fields of mental health where patients are often told that they are 'not sick enough' to qualify for the specialised help that they need. For a patient who has never spoken about the despair of depression to another human being, 12 minutes is a pitiful amount of time. Sometimes it can take that long to utter a sentence.

I'm often asked if I have ever thought of quitting. Well, it has crossed my mind at times, but I don't think that I would walk away. I believe fiercely in what the NHS stands for. I think it is incredible that we can access free health care at the point of delivery. My current trainee, who qualified overseas, is gobsmacked at what the NHS provides. We must protect this.

Global crises like the Covid-19 pandemic force change, and in that confusion and uncertainty there is a space to consider what we want the next step to be. Let's work together to achieve this.

Chapter 4
What does a GP do in today's Britain?

The state of play today is strained for general practice. Everyone has an opinion, but let's look at the data. Huge thanks to Dr Stephen Taylor, a GP with DAUK, for helping me bring these numbers together. He has worked hard since the pandemic compiling facts and figures from various reliable sources, to objectively illustrate what is going on within the NHS. You can follow his posts on X (formerly Twitter)[65] where he provides regular updates on the state of UK general practice.

General practice in 2023 – facts and figures

Some of the key issues affecting general practice at the time of writing in 2023 are outlined below. The BMA updates their workforce statistics every month and you can see current figures here: <www.bma.org.uk/advice-and-support/nhs-delivery-and-workforce>.

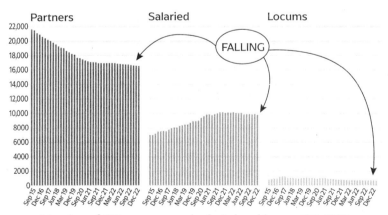

Number of GP partners, and salaried and locum GPs FTE September 2015 to January 2023 *(From the BMA (2023)[1])*

Comparison of historical trends in fully qualified GP numbers (headcount) per 100,000 people in England, with Conservative Party manifesto commitment *(From The Nuffield, Billy Palmer)*

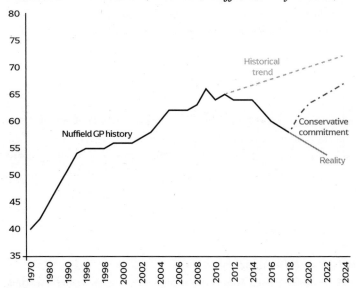

Not enough GPs

Health secretaries regularly promise to recruit more GPs. In 2015, Jeremy Hunt promised 5,000 new GPs in practice by 2020; in 2019 Matt Hancock promised 6,000 by 2023. As of May 2023, we had 2,165 fewer fully qualified full-time GPs compared to September 2015, when data collection began.[66]

The gain in GPs from the year 2000 was steadily lost over the 13 years that followed. In 2022 alone, the NHS lost 402 GP partners alongside 244 salaried, locum and retainer GPs (646 total). Alongside this, the number of GP practices nationwide is falling. This is sometimes due to mergers, but many practices close if they are unable to recruit staff, or if partners retire or die.

Even if the government managed to recruit the promised numbers of GP trainees, this doesn't solve the workforce problem if retention is poor. GPs are leaving the service, and not only those nearing retirement, but the under-30 age group are also walking away. In the 12 months to March 2022, 20.6 per cent of the under thirties workforce left the service[67] – a particularly worrying trend.

**GPs leaving the NHS by age group, full-time equivalent,
September 2016 to June 2022**
*(Reproduced with permission from: N. Davies et al., Performance Tracker
2022, Institute for Government, 2022, www.instituteforgovernment.org.
uk/performance-tracker-2022/general-practice)*

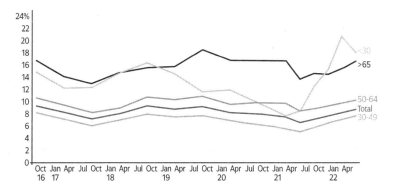

Increased demand

As GP numbers have fallen, the number of registered patients at GP practices has risen by 7 per cent since 2016 to over 62 million. This translates to each GP caring for 2,305 patients (19 per cent more than in 2015).[68]

During winter of 2021, appointment bookings in general practice reached record highs, and levels continue to remain high. Figures from 2022 show GP teams were seeing 10 per cent of the population each week, with 1.4 million appointments per day recorded. This did not include Covid vaccination appointments or account for the long list of other work GPs were also doing. It is likely that the actual number of consultations GPs were doing in this period was much higher than these reported figures, because those done online and or via text are new ways of working since 2019, and these are not captured and counted in these figures.

This number reflects a 20 per cent rise since 2019, and actually more of these were face to face than pre-pandemic. In 2019, 80 per cent of appointments were face to face (actual number 960,000) and in 2022, 70 per cent were face to face but in actual numbers this was 980,000 appointments. In fact, we are seeing more patients face to face now than we were in 2019, and this is alongside all the extra telephone and online consults.[69]

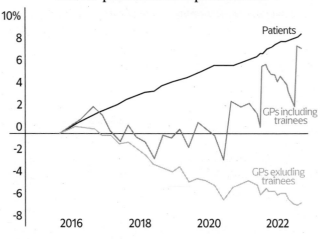

Change in GP numbers and patients registered with GP practices since September 2015

Less funding

In the year 2021–2, NHS GP practices in England were paid £163.65 per registered patient for their care for the year.[70] This amounted to just over £10 billion across 6,758 general practice service providers.[71] To give this some context, the failed NHS test and trace service rapidly established in 2020 to help prevent the spread of Covid, was allocated a budget of £37 billion over 2 years (about 20 per cent of the NHS's entire annual budget).[72]

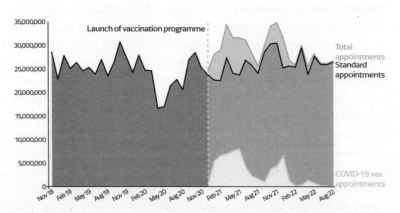

Appointments in General Practice including COVID-19 vaccinations
November 2018 to August 2022

Publication coverage
Details of which GP activities are included,
partially included or not included in the publication.

Included
- scheduled surgery appointments
- scheduled telephone consultations

The following activities are partially included, if they are in the GP system as individual appointments and booked to a patient
- telephone triage
- online consultations
- home visits
- immunisations
- extended access appointments

Face to face	16,949,411
Home visit	187,690
Telephone	7,973,209
Video/Online	143,607
Unknown mode	660,138

Not included
- administration
- supervision
- consultation activity not booked via appointment systems
- training
- meetings
- paperwork
- contacting specialists
- teaching
- prescriptions: reviewing
- prescriptions: actions and results
- running the business
- dealing with complaints
- complying with regulation
- processing laboratory tests
- cancelled appointments that were not rebooked

Hospital waiting lists
Covid significantly impacted service delivery in secondary care, causing backlogs which will take years to clear. Pre-pandemic, there were already 4.43 million people waiting for care – but by June 2023, this figure had rocketed to over 7.5 million. The median waiting time for treatment rose over the same period from 7.2 weeks to 14.3 weeks.[73] Certain mental health services now have a 2-year wait.[74] These patients still require care, and this falls again on general practice.

Newspaper headlines have squarely blamed GPs for driving up the presentations to emergency departments, but the figures, once again, tell the true story. Attendance to A&E is actually no higher than pre-pandemic levels – it is the same story with 999 and 111 calls. It is waiting times that have shot up. And more people are waiting over 12 hours for a decision regarding admission. Ambulance queues are long. Patient flow through hospitals is hampered by the lack of beds. And 'bed blocking' is happening because of the lack of space in social care.[75, 76]

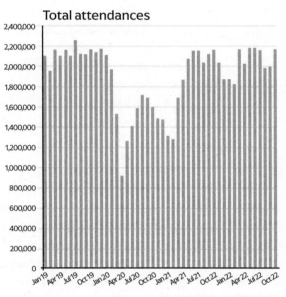

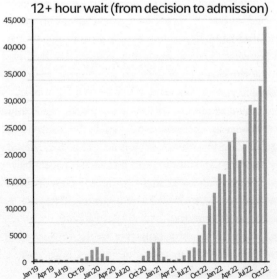

NHS emergency department attendances and waits in England January 2019 to October 2022

Calls, incidents, convey to ED, England, per day
The numbers of incidents per day (21,820) and incidents
with conveyance to ED per day (11,104) in October 2022 were
fewer than in all months from June 2020 to July 2022 inclusive.

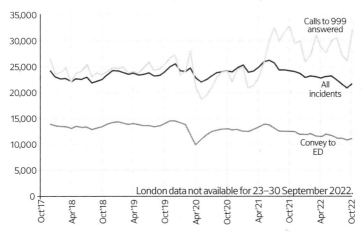

Working patterns

Part-time GPs are the root of all these problems, according to the commentators. Since 2017, the number of GPs working full-time hours or more clinically has been decreasing. We do ourselves a disservice in general practice by the way we describe our working hours in 'sessions'. A GP session is defined as 4 hours 10 minutes. But the reality is, this has stretched to become often more than 6 hours.[77] This means that on paper we are part timers, but we are generally working additional unpaid hours just to get through the workload.

The 2021 GP Worklife Survey showed that the average GP worked 6.3 sessions a week, which should equate to 26.25 hours by the classic definition of a session.[78] This translates as part time. However, the survey also found that the average number of hours GPs worked each week was 38.4 hours per week (12.15 hours extra than the definition of 6.3 sessions). This imbalance between working hours and contracted hours does not account for the additional 50 hours of personal time doctors are meant to assign each year to CPD and keeping up to date on developments in medicine.

Workforce surveys show GP working hours per week:
- 80 per cent of GPs are working over 35 hours
- 60 per cent of GPs are working over 40 hours

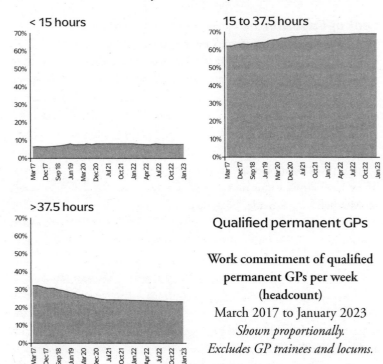

Qualified permanent GPs

Work commitment of qualified permanent GPs per week (headcount)
March 2017 to January 2023
Shown proportionally.
Excludes GP trainees and locums.

- 24 per cent of GPs are working over 50 hours
- 9 per cent of GPs are working over 60 hours[79]

Getting an appointment

An NHS England survey carried out between January and April 2023 asked 759,143 patients their experiences of booking a GP appointment.[80] Less than half of the patients surveyed reported that they found it easy to get through to their GP surgery on the telephone (49.8 per cent) and only half reported a good experience when they did. Getting an appointment proved difficult for 15.9 per cent, either because no appointment was offered, or they couldn't take the slot offered to them. The survey reported that 12.2 per cent of patients who could not secure a GP appointment went to emergency departments for care. The quality of care provided by GPs was rated high by 83.8 per cent, and 91 per cent of patients said their needs had been met.

Fear of litigation

Medical defence organisation, the Medical Protection Society (MPS), surveyed their members back in 2017.[81] They found that 84 per cent of over 1,300 UK GPs stated that the fear of being sued led to them ordering more tests or referrals. They say a full-time GP can expect to receive two clinical negligence claims over their career, and while patients who suffer serious long-term harm due to clinical negligence should be reasonably compensated, there is a growing trend to claim for minor injuries.

Some prominent cases over recent years have impacted the profession. These have implications on the way GPs practice. The 2022 Toombes vs Mitchell[82] case made legal history, when disability activist Evie Toombes, who was born with a neural tube defect, successfully sued her mother's GP, Dr Philip Mitchell, arguing that she would never have been conceived had her mother been given adequate pre-conceptual advice on the benefits of folic acid supplements. The case centred on the documentation in what would have been a 10-minute consultation carried out over 20 years ago. Dr Mitchell wrote 'folate if desired' in the notes and described his usual practice was to give mothers the evidence and let them decide. Mrs Toombes argued this advice was inadequate and she left with the impression she didn't need to take it, and if the advice had been stronger, she would have delayed conception, which would have resulted in a genetically different child.

Aside from the message this sends people with a disability, how does this impact the way doctors now practise? To cover the risks and benefits of every single aspect of care, and to document it, takes far longer than the time allocated to each consultation, not to mention the concerns of practising purely defensive medicine instead of appropriate medicine.

Fear of the regulators

The General Medical Council (GMC) is the regulator for doctors in the UK. It sets the standards that doctors must follow, oversees education and training, and manages a register of doctors who are qualified to practise. The GMC also investigates serious concerns and complaints raised against doctors. It is only right that GPs are held accountable when patients are placing their wellbeing in their hands. GPs make mistakes. Some even break the law. So the medical profession needs a regulator who can uphold standards and enable the public to trust them. However, there have been a slew of cases in recent years which have led doctors to question if the GMC is fit for purpose.

Dr Manjula Arora, a GP in Manchester, was referred to the GMC by her employer Mastercall, for 'dishonesty' over a laptop computer. The case centred around the language used in an exchange between Dr Arora and her medical director. Dr Arora had requested a new work laptop and was told: 'I will note your interest [for] when the next rollout happens.' She later told the IT department over the phone that she had been 'promised' a laptop by the medical director. The representative for the GMC, who chose to pursue the case, accused Dr Arora of lying by saying she had been promised one, saying the wording of her employer was 'entirely unambiguous', and that she had 'brought the profession into disrepute'.[83]

The fact that this case reached the level of a GMC investigation is a travesty. One would hope that even within an organisation, a misinterpretation over some office equipment could be resolved at the local level. But Dr Arora's fitness to practise was questioned and she was suspended from the medical register for 1 month.

A GMC investigation can take anywhere between a few months to years to complete, leaving doctors in professional limbo. Between January 2018 and December 2020, 29 doctors died while under investigation by the GMC. Five of these were confirmed as suicide.[84] We also know that compared with white doctors, those from ethnic minorities are twice as likely to be referred to the GMC by their employers for concerns over fitness to practise. The referral rate among GPs qualifying outside of the UK is three times higher than that among doctors who qualified in the UK.[85] Dr Arora trained in India before moving to the UK in the 1990s.

As GPs, we pay the GMC significant sums of money each year to carry out their role, and we expect a just, proportionate system. When a case, such as this, rears its head, where a doctor poses no risk of harm to patients or the profession, but faces career and life-altering sanctions, it is yet another blow to morale. Can we trust the GMC to protect us from false or malicious complaints? For many, the mistrust is just another reason to leave the profession.

The GMC eventually apologised to Dr Arora for their handling of her case and admitted it should have been resolved locally by Mastercall.[86]

What do the GPs say?

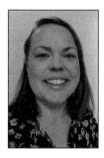

On the pressures

Lizzie Toberty is a GP in Newcastle and GP lead with DAUK. This piece originally appeared in The Times *and is reproduced with permission.*[87]

I have been a GP in the northeast of England for almost 5 years now. In that short time, I have seen a marked decline in the ability of the NHS to provide effective care for patients.

I have seen a growth in the frustration and the depression that goes along with prolonged waits for investigations and operations on the NHS. I have filled out fit notes for years for the same patients, who are awaiting knee and hip replacements, unable to work or move on, with their lives on hold.

I have seen an increase in patients with suspected cancer wait way more than the advised 2 weeks for investigations to either confirm or reassure their worst fears. I have listened to their completely understandable anxious thoughts, unable to offer full reassurance.

I have seen patients with complex mental health problems struggle to get appointments and treatments via the mental health teams, their homes and family lives breaking down as a consequence.

I used to always wait for an ambulance for an unwell patient in the practice if I felt they needed to go to hospital. I knew if I rang 999, an ambulance would usually be with us in about 20 minutes, ensuring safe care of that patient on their way to A&E. Now, if there is any other way of getting them to hospital, for instance a relative could drive them, or a taxi, I have to take the risk, knowing that we could be waiting 4 hours or more for transport.

I have seen patients having prolonged hospital admissions, and sometimes being discharged only to be immediately readmitted because of unsuitable social care arrangements. My colleagues in hospital and care homes are clearly overwhelmed as well. All of the above was relatively uncommon in 2017, when I started. This is now the norm, part of my day-to-day working life.

I empathise, I write seemingly meaningless letters to try to expedite appointments, but I refuse to personally apologise for problems that are not of my making. We, as GPs and health professionals, for too long have stood in the gap between lack of resources and patient needs. We have put our heads down, worked harder and longer. But we cannot do it anymore. We are tired.

It is really tiring trying to provide a service to patients who you know deserve better and to continue to work in a service where poor care is being normalised. We are providing over a million appointments a day with 1,850 fewer doctors than we had in 2015. This number is set to be about 8,800 fewer by 2030 unless there is a significant change in policy. And yet a million appointments a day is not enough. Patient satisfaction is at an all-time low.

There are plenty of opportunities for GPs elsewhere. Adverts for private work, which I never would have considered as a fresh-faced junior doctor, appear on my social media stream all the time.

The ability to control my workload, give the right amount of time to a patient to help them and then get home to see my daughter to bed looks more and more tempting each week. Indeed, some of my colleagues already have started working privately, and report how much their wellbeing has improved.

Most GPs want to work in the NHS, providing free health care. But it is no longer compatible with a long-term healthy and sustainable career. This job is making us ill. This is reflected in the high numbers of doctors who refer themselves for mental health support to the Practitioner Health Programme.

We are human beings and we do have a limit. That is why it is so disappointing to see soundbites, rather than well-thought-out policy, and targets rather than resources. What we have seen is not a developed, considered plan to save the NHS. It represents on-the-hoof thinking by a government that does not have any idea what the actual cause of the access problems are. Most of the ideas have already been tried.

Ministers seem to develop plans without actually speaking to any GPs, practice nurses or managers. How can we provide meaningful change for patients when those making the policies do not engage with our union, our college or the people 'on the ground'?

I am left wondering: is this yet another incompetent government unable to fully comprehend or tackle the real issues, with a sense of realism and honest conversation about what can actually be provided? Or is it part of a more nefarious plan? I can't decide.

Once again, I would encourage government ministers and all MPs, to come and see us, for their own 'face to face'. Understand what we do and how we do it. We might also be able to offer you some of the solutions too.

On home visits

As the population ages, we have larger numbers of people living with complex healthcare needs. Homes visits by GPs have been an integral part of general practice, supporting these frail patients, and providing a unique insight by seeing patients in their own environments. In the current climate of pressures from all angles, the practicalities of home visiting have raised debate. In November 2019, the conference of England LMCs backed a motion to 'remove the anachronism of home visits from core contract work',[88] the response to which was highly emotive with divided opinions among GPs.

GPs working in short-staffed practices overwhelmed with work, view home visits as an inefficient use of scarce resources. Others feel patients regard them as an entitlement, available for their own convenience. I have certainly made visits to people who had been able to pop to the shops and were in the checkout queue when I was knocking at their door. I've also frequently been asked to visit sick children by parents who have had too many gins to drive. It's interesting to note that a home visit in the private sector costs upward of £250.[89]

There has been a decline in home visiting over the last 50 years, both in the UK and internationally.[90] Not all GPs are convinced of their benefits, while many consider them a vital part of the role.

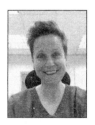

Dr Catriona McNicol is a GP partner in Yorkshire. She wrote this beautiful account of a home visit, illustrating both the pressures and pleasures of seeing patients in their homes.

After a brutal morning surgery, which drew to a close at about 12:59pm, almost 90 minutes later than anticipated, I grabbed a handful of

Celebrations, kindly donated by a patient, and an uber fast, three-gulp cup of tea as a means of sustenance, before packing my bag and heading out on a home visit.

Did I want to go? No. I just wanted to knuckle down and try and work through the mountain of ever-growing tasks and urgent requests that faced me as Duty Doctor. But did I want to help this elderly patient? Yes.

And that's always the conundrum. The wish to actually be there, to be the good old GP, but knowing that the complex home visit won't be a 10-minute job. Time that's just not there, it's an invisible, almost non-existent resource. But we pile on anyway.

So, with a feeling of impending doom about what the afternoon had yet to bring I headed off.

Immediately upon arriving at the address I realised I should have brought a coat as I stood opposite the telecom system which flashed a digital 'service disconnect' message at me.

My skin was rough with goosebumps as I shivered. After 16 minutes I eventually got hold of the patient who came slowly down the many floors to let me in.

We returned to the cosy flat, Christmas cards part written, spread on the small dining room table with festive cheer and obligation.

We consulted. A shared plan was made. I had been there for 15 minutes. So far my visit, including prep, travel time and delay getting into the building, had taken almost 40 minutes.

We wrapped up, and as I was about to leave, my very nearly triple-figure patient looked up hopefully at me and said, 'I know you're very busy, thank you for coming to see me.'

'You're very welcome, it was really lovely to meet you,' I returned, genuinely enthused to have had the opportunity to meet this chap.

'I, eh, well, I don't suppose you would like to see some photos? Do you have time for that?' he asked, eyes wide.

I knew I didn't. Good God, I didn't. I had not a second left to give.

But my heart melted.

'Yes, that would be lovely,' I said as I exhaled, knowing that this was one of those moments. This chap had earned it.

And so we sat and looked at photos of his D-Day landing, talked about that day, I heard of his terrifying introduction to war, and his good fortune in life thereafter, evidenced by the abundance of beautiful, happy family photos I was offered to absorb.

It was only another 15 minutes.

I could have stayed there forever. I pulled myself away. By the time I had returned to the surgery and completed my notes, the whole visit had taken over one hour.

The rest of the day was back breaking.

But tonight, I feel good. I feel lucky. I can't believe I got to hear first-hand from this man what had happened.

Despite getting home at 8pm and feeling absolutely bust, I'm noting this day as a good one.

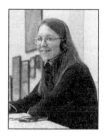

On remote working

I wrote a version of this piece for The Times *in December 2022, and this is reproduced with permission here.[91]*
Copyright Phil Wilkinson Photography and Video

Various newspapers reported with horror this week, the case of a GP working remotely for a practice in Surrey, whilst living over 200 miles away in Cornwall. The comments sections were alight with outrage as keyboard warriors indulged in what has become something of a national sport of late – GP bashing.

The sad irony in all of these articles is that general practice is elbow deep in a recruitment and retention crisis. The obsession with face-to-face appointments from some sections of the media is losing sight of the fact: an experienced remote GP is better than no GP at all.

I'm a remote GP, and I haven't seen a patient face to face since 2019.

I still feel pangs of guilt saying this, despite the fact I manage to clock up at least six sessions a week remotely. In each 4-hour, 10-min session I have 24 patients booked – that's 48 a day – almost double the number of patient contacts the BMA advises is reasonable per day. If someone needs an examination, then I can arrange this with a colleague easily. Patients I consult with are often speaking with me the same day they raise their problem, and many have solutions provided without leaving the comfort of their own homes. The time I spend staring at a screen is increasingly stretched beyond my contracted hours and the work/home boundaries blur as I fit admin in after my children's bedtime.

I'm not unique. Working remotely in any other sector would barely raise an eyebrow. It's a choice I have made, like a million other working mums, to salvage the time spent commuting, to be able to earn if my children get sick and I have no childcare and to enable the juggle. It allowed me to return to NHS work within weeks of having both my children, which I just wouldn't have done otherwise, something I simultaneously regard as a privilege that I could do so and a curse that I didn't have longer simply being a new mum.

Technology has changed the way almost all sectors of our society function. In the year 2000, less than 7 per cent of the world had internet access. Today, over half the global population is online. Similarly with mobile phones, they were a novelty in the 2000s, and now there are over 8 billion mobile phone subscriptions worldwide. There are more mobile phones than there are people.[92] Most people do banking and shopping online. If we go for a supermarket face to face, we see an expanse of self-checkout kiosks rather than a friendly cashier.

However, as a GP, the rules are somehow different. The old-fashioned image of a GP is of a kindly old man with a Gladstone bag, cheerfully popping in for a home visit with his patients at any time of the day or night. This is unrealistic in the world we now live in. The sense of vocation associated with being a GP has sadly been corroded, and nowadays, doctors are qualifying with debts stretching to six figures and tolerating working conditions that are impacting on our mental health. The workload in general practice now is unrecognisable compared to even 10 years ago when I started out. GPs are consulting with more patients than ever before. We're handling the backlog of care from the pandemic and often dealing with patients unable to access secondary care. Remote medicine can be transactional, but it increases efficiency and provides a safety valve to take some of the pressure off a system which is at breaking point. The reality that the headlines also ignore is that many patients also prefer it.

Telemedicine is huge elsewhere in the world and countries such as Australia have embraced it to provide care to remote areas. Even in the UK, specialties such as radiology have been utilising it for years, often employing doctors based overseas to help with their workload. It's convenient, it's safe when done well, and it allows those hard-to-recruit areas to gain access to a doctor they would have otherwise gone without. We also forget that in 2020, remote consulting was mandated by the government. What is interesting, is that video consultations have not really taken off. As Helen Salisbury points out in the *British Medical Journal*,[93] the predicted video revolution never happened with less than 1 per cent of consultations in general practice (in England) being conducted this way in May 2023.[94] The telephone trumps a blurred video for me, and an in-person consult is safer if needed.

The practice I work for in Carlisle, Cumbria, set up a bank of remote GPs to plug long-standing workforce gaps. Several local practices in the county in deprived areas use this GP bank as it helps to stabilise practices that have previously struggled to recruit. In total 33 GPs signed up to the bank, with 10 working regular shifts. This model has allowed the founding practice alone to boost its own workforce with an extra two to three full-time equivalent GPs, adding roughly 15 per cent to its GP capacity.[95]

As GP numbers continue to plummet, those of us who haven't left for double the salary in Australia or the private sector are increasingly burning out. Abuse towards NHS staff is commonplace. The number of doctors dying by suicide is on the rise. The recent death of hardworking GP Dr Gail Milligan (discussed in Chapter 3 'GPs and the pandemic') was attributed directly to her overwhelming workload. Whatever your opinion is on remote working, the simple maths tells us we don't have enough GPs right now. We need to move away from this negative narrative around GPs and applaud creative solutions to bolster the workforce.

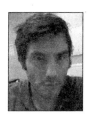

On workload caps

Dr Paul Evans is a GP and chair of Gateshead and South Tyneside Local Medical Committee. He previously served as a British army doctor in Iraq and Afghanistan. This piece first appeared in metro.co.uk in December 2022 and is reproduced here with permission.[96]

I looked up at the clock and it was 7pm.

I'd been in the surgery for 12 hours, spoken to 50 patients, signed 80 prescriptions, checked and acted upon a similar number of lab results and had a meeting with the commissioners about the ongoing lack of space in local surgeries for growing populations.

Within that time, I was sustained only by several lukewarm cups of tea and the odd trip to the toilet. If you were my next patient, how safe would that make you feel?

Well, according to the BMA, seeing more than 25 patients per day leads to decision fatigue and patient safety risks. I ask again: how safe do you feel?

But the above, I'm afraid, is a typical day for many in general medical practice in England. It's what I, and many of my colleagues, feel we have to do in order to get our work done and care for as many of our patients as possible.

That's why I'm calling for GPs to work a standard 8-hour working day.

You might ask, but haven't GPs always worked these hours?

Yes: when the majority were men with stay-at-home wives.

Yes: when the demands were fewer, the medicine less complex and other services (such as mental health services) were functional.

Yes: when the working day started early and finished late, but doctors had permitted time to leave the surgery for fresh air, to catch up with colleagues or simply to eat lunch while not staring at a screen.

The working day of a GP now bears little resemblance to that of as little as a decade ago.

Despite growing numbers of trainee GPs, the number of full-time equivalent GPs falls every year, including crucial partners, which are those who hold contr acts and responsibility for their surgeries. All the while, the population becomes larger, older and more unwell.

In 2015, the Health Secretary at the time, Jeremy Hunt, promised 5,000 new GPs by 2021. Well, where are we now?

Earlier this year, Hunt admitted: 'When I left office...we'd only got an extra 300. And in fact, since then, we've gone backwards, you know, 1,500 fewer GPs. I hold myself completely responsible for the failure to deliver that.'[97]

As partner numbers fall, the GPs who remain increasingly have to juggle a lot more – including cancelled leave, marriages under strain and missed opportunities to see their children grow up. This outlook worsens the outflow of partners and speeds up the death spiral of surgeries.

After all, a surgery in trouble with burnt-out doctors is not one many GPs wish to join.

This is particularly true in light of the tragedy of Dr Gail Milligan.

GPs all over the country recognise the 'Sunday evening log-on' as a regular feature of life, a doomed attempt to mitigate the flood of work on Mondays.

Hand on heart, I do not know a single recently qualified GP who wishes to take up partnership, as they see the toll it takes on their older colleagues. I know far more who have left their partnerships – and their patients – as they simply could not cope any longer with the workload.

This is why I proposed at the England LMC Conference in November 2022 that surgery core opening hours be cut to 8 hours per day, which would be 40 per week. I presume it is why this motion was passed by a majority of the GPs present.[98]

Currently, GPs are usually working when the surgery is open between 8am and 6:30pm, Monday to Friday (52.5 hours per week). These hours are packed non-stop with decision after complex decision, then more hours after the surgery closes to perform necessary administrative work.

But this model is failing doctors and patients alike, creating barriers to younger GPs, who may want to provide quality, continuous care from cradle to grave, but who cannot see a way to make the commitment work with their families.

Women are particularly affected by these working hours because they unfairly shoulder childcare responsibilities. Seriously, try finding childcare that opens longer than 8am to 6pm. Now work out how this is compatible with having young children and a demanding career – it just isn't.

The incoming workforce needs to be able to see a job that they can do safely, without it causing them active harm.

We need NHS leaders to see that making ineffective changes and essentially forcing fewer GPs to work even harder will lead to a future of practices opening long hours but staffed by a succession of non-partnership staff who have little knowledge of their patients.

Do you want 40 hours per week of GPs you know and trust, or 52.5 hours of assorted temporary staff? Which of these do you want for your child, or your elderly relative?

This all sounds very gloomy, I know.

I would be lying if I said general practice is not at a crisis point, but it's salvageable if those in charge are prepared to listen to GPs.

We want them to accept that we wish to do right by our patients, and they should trust that if this simple change is made, then younger GPs – who are currently not willing to commit to long-term work at a practice – will be more likely to do so.

Honestly, the temptation to quit the responsibility of partnership, go locum and set my own hours raises its head frequently. However, I cannot bring myself to walk away from my patients.

I urge you to consider whether a GP workforce that is well-rested, healthy and able to look forward to coming to work is what you wish for, or whether you want more of the same.

BBC File on 4 spent a week at Dr Evans' surgery in Tyneside in July 2023. You can listen to their report here: <www.bbc.co.uk/sounds/play/m001npb4>.

On pay restoration
The junior doctor strikes of 2023 have been the longest period of industrial action taken in the history of the health service and a reflection of the mood of the profession. The consultants hit the picket lines in July 2023, and in April, GPs voted overwhelmingly to ballot for industrial action if 'disastrous' contract changes are not renegotiated.[99] Lizzie Toberty, GP lead with DAUK tells us why doctors are voting with their feet.

When it comes to doctors' pay, we're asking the wrong questions. The junior doctors' strikes of 2023 prompted health commentators to ask if doctors are paid too much or too little, and if they should be allowed pension tax breaks, or not?

A debate raged through the profession following a BMA advert in the *Guardian*, questioning comparisons between the pay of Pret baristas and junior doctors. Doctors, both new school and old school, MPs, unions and plenty of commentators jumped into the discussion.

⊕BMA The BMA
@TheBMA

Full page in @guardian today. Let's spread the word about #payrestoration for Junior Doctors

#DayTwo #JuniorDoctorsStrike

PRET A MANGER HAS ANNOUNCED IT WILL PAY UP TO £14.10 PER HOUR. A JUNIOR DOCTOR MAKES JUST £14.09.

THANKS TO THIS GOVERNMENT YOU CAN MAKE MORE SERVING COFFEE THAN SAVING PATIENTS

The degree is gruelling, the job near impossible to get right, the debt astronomical and the postgraduate training enough to strain even the most well suited of relationships. There is a huge personal cost to being a doctor.

Despite this, is it morally right for doctors to demand pay restoration? Should a weekly clap on the doorstep be enough? Is medicine a vocation rather than a job?

Should highly qualified people accept lower wages in the public sector to serve the greater good?

It seems everyone, not least doctors themselves, has been getting tied in knots, trying to justify their position.

The current Health Secretary, Steve Barclay, advised doctors to 'check their conscience'. Things really are at a low when emotional blackmail is used in an attempt to stabilise the workforce.

But really, though, we're asking the wrong questions.

The really important question we all need to be asking is, 'If I get ill, do I want a doctor to be available, free at the point of access, to treat me?' Remember, the longer we wait for both emergency and routine care, the poorer the outcome.

The reality is we do not have enough doctors. There are thousands of vacancies across the NHS, and despite expanded medical schools and postgraduate training programmes, those vacancies are not getting filled. Doctors are moving abroad, reducing hours, moving to the private sector or retiring early. Whether you like it or not, this is the reality. With each doctor who moves that's one less to treat you or your family.

No amount of telling workers in any sector they should just put up with their lot will help expand a workforce. Improving conditions and pay will.

The last decade has seen huge advances in all aspects of medicine – life changing drugs for patients with cystic fibrosis, incredible treatments curing and prolonging the lives of cancer patients and huge leaps in outcomes for pre-term babies, to name a few. We are getting better all the time at keeping people alive.

It follows, though, we need a workforce capable to deliver these complex treatments and look after those patients when they survive.

We have a government who stand for market forces and capitalism. This is what is playing out now, globally. There is a shortage of workers which the international market is more than happy to bid for. But for some reason, we believe the 'privilege' of working in the NHS should mean workers should just put up with their lot and the UK should not need to compete on the world stage. It's incongruent with our wider attitude to economic growth.

Consequently, healthcare providers from Australia are flying over to run recruitment events, tempting doctors over with better conditions, and salaries three times what is offered in the UK. I calculated that

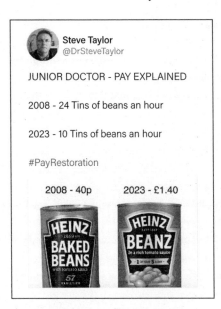

Steve Taylor
@DrSteveTaylor

JUNIOR DOCTOR - PAY EXPLAINED

2008 - 24 Tins of beans an hour

2023 - 10 Tins of beans an hour

#PayRestoration

2008 - 40p   2023 - £1.40

with 3 years in Australia as a GP I could probably pay my mortgage off.

Every time I read an article by a political commentator stating doctors are greedy, or a retired consultant harking on that back in their day they never slept and were paid £100 a week, I feel a little more undervalued and the antipodes, where well-paid work awaits, looks more appealing. If I was in my twenties, without children, I would almost certainly be there right now.

So, I say, whatever your thoughts about greedy doctors, pay restoration or pension allowances, put them aside. Ask yourself this: 'Next time I'm sick, do I want a doctor to be freely available to me?'

If the answer is yes, then we need to work out a way to pay for them. We can't afford not to.

Key facts on pay restoration[100]

Junior doctors are qualified doctors who are on a training pathway to become a generalist (GP) or a specialist. This training can take anything from 5–11 years. Since 2008, junior doctors have seen a 26 per cent real terms pay cut. The basic pay of a first year (foundation) doctor in England is £29,384 a year for full time (40 hours) weekday working. Additional pay may be received for unsocial and additional hours. This equates to a basic hourly pay of £14.09 per hour. The Junior Doctors Committee (JDC) of the doctors' union of the BMA called on the government to restore junior doctor pay in England to its 2008–9 levels – an uplift of around 35 per cent. The government did not engage, prompting several rounds of industrial action by junior doctors.[101]

On the 10-minute consult

There is a quote in Polly Morland's *A Fortunate Woman*[102] which rings true. A patient talking about her GP says: 'The point is, she's a person not a service. That's why she's always late for appointments. It's because she's spent time with the one before you. And, if you ask me, that's a very good thing.'

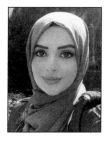

GP Dr Zainab Batool captures the essence of time pressures in her journal, on the way home from a 'normal' GP day.

This was my 'last straw' day, the '10-minute tragedy' that is GP appointments.

This was after a decade of hospital shifts, trying to reach this 'finish line'. It was after reading for years in tabloids that GPs do nothing much and hearing this rhetoric back from patients.

Deep breath.
Clear the last patients from my mind, for now.
The angry, the sad.
Wipe away.
Smile wide.
Screw tired eyes shut.
Shrug away the back pain.
Need to pee, maybe after the next three.
Change PPE.

Next patient please.
Scroll through notes, blood tests, letters, scans.
'Didn't you read my notes?' said one. Yes, but I didn't know which of 16 problems you were coming for. Please don't shout. Wipe away.

2 mins:
He is shuffling down the corridor, knees aren't what they were. He's dressed in his Sunday best, white hair combed neatly to one side.

Stand to greet, smile wider, here I am, how can I help?

'Oh, just a few things,' he says.

Heartsink, deep breath. I'll do what I can, can't say no when he asks so nicely.

His chest hurts and he bleeds when he goes to the toilet. He can't sleep and he wakes up with a headache. Just a few red flags, that's all. Must sort. When, where, how long? Winding stories, family anecdotes. Smile wide.

I'm sorry the hospital delayed the appointment. Can I speed it up? Probably not. I'm very sorry, very sorry. I can try.

12 mins:

Let's pop you on the couch to examine.

Layers of clothes and arthritis.

Let me help. Hope that didn't sound hasty.

Dr, could you just take a look at my nails while you're here?

18 mins:

4 patients waiting.

I know I'm very sorry, very sorry.

Printer out of prescription paper. I'll just pop out, won't be long.

There's a glaring crowd at reception. Deep breath.

Sorry.

Doc, could you please sign this while you're here?

Of course.

Smile wide.

Look down. Don't meet the angry eyes.

Don't smile too wide.

I haven't stopped, I promise.

I'm trying my best, I promise.

I miss my kids.

Here I am Sir, back again, sorry to keep you.

23 mins:

Take care, goodbye.

Nice to meet you.

Please don't complain.

Please don't get more sick.

Type hard and fast.
Mustn't forget a word.
Would it stand in court?
Dear hospital, pls see Mr P earlier even though I know you can't.
I'll order the bloods at night from laptop.
Cancer referral now though.

29 mins:

Next patient please.
'Hello little one,' smile wide.
Out of stickers.
Miss my kids.
Won't see them before they sleep.
'We've been waiting an hour you know.'
I know.
I'm sorry.
Sorry for my best.
Need to pee.
I miss my kids.
I want to go home.
Wipe away, smile wide.
I'm very sorry.
Here I am, how can I help?

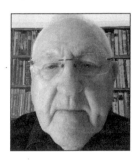

What do the patients think?

Ron Templeton is a retired academic tutor. He spent many years tutoring generations of medical students at Liverpool Medical School and describes his experiences as both a patient and a tutor.

I was born in February 1940, 8 years before the foundation of the NHS. My knowledge of general practice goes back to those pre-NHS days when as a boy I remember visiting the family doctor's surgery, which was a room in his own house.

The waiting room had a row of seats, a central coffee table containing out-of-date magazines and a one bar electric fire. He would give me potions he had concocted himself. On occasions he would do a house call and my mother would provide a dessert spoon and a shilling for his services. Thankfully those primitive days have long gone, and surgeries are now state of the art with piped music and pictures of 'The Team'. However, these state-of-the-art practices don't seem enough to attract young doctors. I am sad to hear so many complaints by friends and family about their experiences with their GP practices these days. As a patient, I have been lucky with the treatment and service I receive. I tend not to go too often to my GP, unless absolutely necessary, and I try not to overdo the consultation. However, like many patients, I'm not very happy with telephone consultations as it's impersonal. What happened to examination as part of a diagnosis?

From an early age I wanted to be a doctor. However, in the 1950s if you didn't get your A-levels first time then that meant no university. I settled for the pathology labs.

When I started as a tutor at the Liverpool Medical School the problem-based learning (PBL) course was introduced as a perceived stepping-stone to general practice – encouraging problem solving and independent learning. Sadly, we now have less trainees entering general practice.

I spent 15 years as both an academic and personal tutor at Liverpool Medical School working with medical students from the first year up to final year and often postgraduates too, gaining their thoughts on placements both in hospitals and general practices. My recollections were that they were not always given doctor contact but encouraged to sit in with practice nurses and the wider practice team to gain an understanding of how the whole system worked. I personally felt the way to attract further family practitioners, was for students to spend more time with the GPs themselves, to see at first-hand what GPs do. Maybe the perceived lack of enthusiasm by GPs is a contributory factor to why general practice is not so attractive.

Although there was an excellent Community Studies Unit of the Liverpool School of Medicine, supporting around 140 GP tutors to provide clinical placements for student doctors in years 2, 3, 4 and 5, there was not much time to carry out other projects involving general practices. I would think that general practice would be attractive to young doctors for the following reasons: no on call; no weekend or bank holiday work; practice managers to run the practice; probably less hassle and bullying than in hospitals; and reasonable pay. (*Note from the author: GPs do work on call and do out-of-hours weekend and bank holiday work. Many GPs working as partners manage their own practices, including resolving HR issues. The average GP pay ranges from £64,900 for salaried GPs to £142,000 for contractor GPs in England as of 2020–21.*[103])

Television programmes like 'GPs Behind Closed Doors' should help recruitment. So why are young medics not attracted to general practice? I believe radio, television and social media have not helped the reputation of the profession; day after day there are complaints about the lack of service. They trot out the usual complaints: can't get an appointment, have to wait a week or more; rude and unhelpful receptionists; can't see the same doctor each time; no face-to-face appointments – the lists go on and on. This adverse publicity cannot help recruitment, even if it is based in truth.

If I were starting out on a medical career, I would certainly be put off choosing general practice because of the continued hammering and bad publicity in the press, especially newspapers, of how bad GPs are. Attacking the profession for remote consultations, labelling them as lazy, work shy, not bothering to turn up for work. All this has had a knock-on effect involving the general public who have joined in the fore and have, in some cases, not only verbally, but physically attacked practice staff including doctors and receptionists. The government seems to be uninterested and has not intervened. It is not surprising that those working in general practice are fed up with the situation and are voting with their feet.

Increased workload with little thanks; increased number of patients per practice due to closures of near-by surgeries; increased paperwork at the end of each surgery: prescriptions, letters, diagnostic tests interpretation, restricted time restraints in seeing patients.

The erosion of the unique relationship between family doctors and their patients has left many GPs wondering why they are in the profession.

Chapter 5
Does it work better elsewhere?

Medicine is a global profession and judging from the exodus of UK-trained doctors to work overseas, life really is better as a doctor elsewhere. The 2022 GMC workforce report showed that 4,843 doctors left the UK to work overseas between May 2021 and May 2022,[104] while a BMA survey from the same year found that four in 10 doctors surveyed planned to leave the NHS as soon as they could find another job – a third of these hoped to move abroad, with Australia and Canada listed as the top destinations.[105]

The UK is now falling behind the rest of the world, both in terms of staffing and equipment.

And more worryingly, the NHS has higher avoidable mortality rates, with below-average survival rates for many cancers. The UK spends less per person on health than both Australia and Canada (and France, Denmark, the Netherlands, Germany, and many others).[106] Is it any wonder people are going elsewhere?

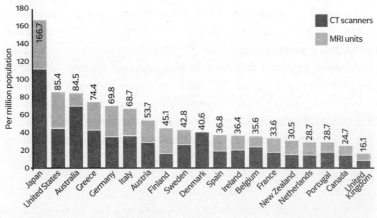

The UK has fewer CT and MRI scanners than comparator countries
CTI and MRI scanners per million head of population,
2019 or nearest year

The UK has fewer doctors and nurses per head than most of its peers
Practising doctors and nurses, selected countries, 2019
(Taken from https://www.kingsfund.org.uk/blog/2023/06/comparing-nhs-health-care-systems-other-countries-five-charts)

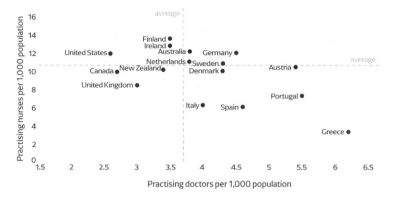

In this chapter we hear from doctors who have made the move. They tell us just what it is like in health systems outside the NHS. We hear from an emergency medicine consultant with experience working in four different countries who explains just why things are so bad in the NHS and how doctors are valued elsewhere. A Merseyside GP who moved to Canada tells us the differences she has experienced, while a Norwegian GP tells us how their health system is not that different from the NHS. A GP who ran her own practice in New Zealand and returned to the UK describes how we can learn from the system down under to improve things here. I describe my time on cruise ships and the dangers of a fee-paying model.

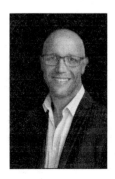

Anywhere is better than the NHS

After 12 years of brutal NHS service, Dr Neil Barnard left his post as an emergency department consultant to work abroad in 2022. He told me his reasons for this decision. Excerpts from an opinion piece Dr Barnard wrote for metro.co.uk, are reproduced with permission here. [107]

'I was tired and had little more left to give to the NHS,' said Barnard. 'I drove to work each day, without the sense of anticipation I had earlier in my career. Instead, I had a feeling of foreboding that the day would bring issues over which I had no control, precipitated by years of under-investment and service cuts alongside criminally poor investment in adult social care services.'

Dr Barnard has worked around the globe. Born and trained in South Africa, he came to the UK in 2010 on a Tier 2 working visa, after working in Australia and having had a stint on cruise ships. He obtained a British passport in 2014. He completed 8 years of specialist training in the UK (in both emergency and intensive care medicine) and then moved with his family, for a 2-year sabbatical in New Zealand. Taking a step away from the UK system highlighted just how bad things had become within the NHS, and although he did return to an NHS consultant post after his time in the antipodes, the seed was planted to make the move more permanent.

The value placed upon doctors was the most striking difference that Neil observed, comparing the approach taken towards doctors in New Zealand and the NHS.

> *My New Zealand starting salary was £115,000 per year. I would need to remain in the NHS as a consultant for 19 years to achieve parity.[108] All my professional fees were paid by my trust. I was afforded a relocation allowance of £10,000 and given a generous educational budget of £7,500.*

Doctors are required to stay up to date and meet certain standards to revalidate their medical licences. In the UK this study is typically done in personal time, often crammed in around brutal rotas. Emergency medics are also required to stay up to date with at least three life-support training courses which are delivered over 2–3 days of intensive training. Barnard is a teacher on all three of these courses and in order to maintain his teaching status, he needs to teach on a total of six courses a year. 'In the UK,' he says, 'I need to undertake this teaching commitment in my private time. In New Zealand, there is an understanding that this training is essential to ensure quality patient care, and teaching leave is granted to ensure this happens.'

'There are many more hidden costs to being a doctor that the public don't see,' adds Barnard, 'I hold professional registration in four countries. I am a fellow of three specialist faculties and hold membership of an educational academy.'

> *All these fees are mandatory and cost in excess of £3,000. I am obliged to hold private indemnity insurance which, as an emergency medicine consultant with responsibility for a large group of junior staff, amounts to a further £1,500 annually. Continuing professional development, mandated by the GMC costs yet more, and we can't forget the exorbitant NHS car parking fees. This amounts to thousands of pounds a year. In New Zealand, all of this is covered by the hospital. Junior doctors get a hot meal every day for free, with more mandatory rest periods, more annual leave and non-clinical time to allow work on other projects. Work-life balance is valued.*

Compare these perks to what is on offer for doctors coming to work in the UK from overseas, which is a costly, bureaucratic process. In 2015, the coalition government introduced the Immigration Health Surcharge (IHS), which is an annual fee of £624 that migrants need to pay to use the NHS. For a family of four, this charge, along with visa fees, can easily reach £10,000 a year, which for tax paying NHS staff is an extortionate amount of money to have to pay to access the very system they work within (and ultimately pay for twice). In October 2020, a small perk was granted when the Prime Minister announced that international health and care staff and their dependants would be exempt from the IHS, in view of their efforts during the pandemic.

'The process in the UK was expensive,' recalls Barnard, 'but relatively straightforward as I held an internationally recognised medical degree and was married to a UK national. I did, however, find it illogical that I was required to pay for and sit the mandatory International English Language Test System (IELTS) exam, given that my first language is English. Making the move to New Zealand was a lot simpler and the perks on offer were incomparable.'

Barnard's decision to leave the NHS wasn't purely financial. The below-inflation pay rises offered to healthcare staff, combined with the cost-of-living crisis, was certainly a factor. 'I don't feel I am being adequately compensated for the years of training, hard work and sacrifice I have endured in order to become a senior specialist in not one but two specialties,' he said. However, he adds, 'I can no longer face the fact that I can't do the job I am trained to do because the system doesn't support me doing it.'

> *Emergency departments need to deal with the sickest patients quickest. In order to do this, we need space to assess and diagnose the patient, staff to attend to them and equipment to cater for their needs. Very often, the beds we have are filled with patients waiting to go to the wards.*
>
> *The wards have no space because their beds are filled with patients awaiting residential or nursing home placement. The evidence is unequivocal that long waits in A&E are associated with increased mortality,[109] yet, our patients continue to suffer as we treat them in corridors and inappropriate non-clinical spaces while ambulances are stacked outside waiting to hand over new patients.[110]*

Barnard's exit strategy has involved working for a telemedicine company in Australia. 'It is a travesty that it's easier for me to write an after-hours prescription for Shane in Kalgoorlie than it is to provide the same service for Ahmad in Kettering.'

> *I could never leave medicine – I love the work and I find it a privilege to treat patients. I can no longer work in a system that hamstrings its staff, undervalues us and does not look after our long-term health and wellbeing. When staff are crying as a result of the workload and the stress of the job, the answer is not to be forced to undertake mandatory resilience training in our spare time.*
>
> *The NHS needs to realise that its staff is its greatest asset. More than the buildings and theatres, it's the staff that keep the service going. For years, staff have gone above and beyond the call of duty out of a sense of pride or obligation to keep the service afloat. Now, with Covid having tested the limits of our endurance and brought into focus the priority of time and family, the goodwill bank is running dry. NHS workers are suffering from Stockholm Syndrome. We are in an abusive relationship but have become enthralled to our abuser. Many of us have not had our eyes opened to the way we deserve to be treated and the way a system should and could function.*
>
> *I am sad to leave my friends and colleagues in the NHS, many of whom are some of the finest people I've ever had the privilege to*

work with. I have no doubt, if conditions fail to improve within the NHS, I will work with many of them again – only this time in warmer climes and with stranger accents.

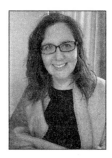

From Merseyside
to Nova Scotia

Dr Sarah Rushworth is a GP in Nova Scotia, Canada, who made the move from her NHS job in Merseyside in 2021.

There was never a moment when I definitely thought I had to leave the NHS. Our move to Canada happened very insidiously, and because of all the paperwork, it was completed over such a long time-frame that it just crept up on me. Initially my head was turned by the promise of more money when a recruiter reached out to me back in February 2019. At the time I was just starting out as a locum GP, having left a 5-year salaried position. My husband had his dream job, and our oldest child was settled at school. A move to Canada seemed exciting but not practical.

Life as a locum continued and I was offered a partnership at a practice where I was covering maternity leave. The partnership starting date was quicker than I had anticipated and occurred just at the start of the pandemic in April 2020. It is difficult to say how the pandemic impacted my experience of partnership, or whether I was simply tired of relentless phone triage, increased workload and dissatisfied patients. This is when I decided to make enquiries about working in Canada.

In September 2020, I started to complete the multiple forms needed, every step of the way thinking that the College of Physicians and Surgeons, Nova Scotia, may turn around and say, 'no' to me, but they didn't. By March 2021, I had an offer of a full licence to practise and could apply for a work permit. Again, this was more paperwork, but the permit was agreed at the beginning of July 2021, and we booked our flights. During the entire process I had decided that despite committing to working in Canada, I wanted to ensure I didn't lose my licence to practice in the UK. I continued to ensure I was meeting all the criteria needed to stay on the UK Performers List, remaining registered with the GMC and continuing with my appraisals and revalidation.

Arriving in Canada was quite a culture shock. We arrived, as a family of four (my husband; son, aged 7; and daughter, aged 3) with four suitcases and the promise of a shipping container which was due to arrive in 2 months. We had accommodation booked for 2 weeks due to Covid regulations as the children needed to quarantine, but then we needed to find somewhere to live after that. There was a lot to organise and contend with as well as starting work. I had to finish my registration documents, open a bank account, get a car and insurance, find somewhere to live and enrol the children in school, just to name a few. The support from the Nova Scotia Health Authority in doing this was absent and we relied on the good will and advice of other doctors from the UK and my new practice manager who was fantastic.

We muddled through, and 2 weeks after arriving I started my new practice in Cole Harbour. I was starting from scratch, which meant I had to build a patient list (panel) from the beginning and had to learn to negotiate my way around a new electronic medical records (EMR) system and the intricacies of referring to secondary care.

There are currently 100,000 people in Nova Scotia without a family physician, so demand for a GP is huge. Many patients have not had a regular doctor for years and have relied on walk-in clinics, emergency rooms and the good will of hospital physicians to fill their regular prescriptions and manage problems outside their remit. The waiting times to be seen in the emergency room are often long, usually due to the patients having no access to a family physician and having nowhere else to go. There is no referral pathway to a dedicated medical or surgical assessment unit for those that have urgent problems and need to be seen same day but are not accidents or emergencies. There is an urgent need for family physicians in Nova Scotia and this was something I did not appreciate when I was applying to come here. There is a lot of inequality. There are very limited private health services available in the province and these have been relatively new additions. Previously, even if you had money and wanted to pay for services, you were unable to do so.

I can honestly say I have never been welcomed so warmly. Some patients would cry when they met me for the first time as they had not had a family doctor in years, others thanked me profusely for coming to their country and expressed their gratitude that I was leaving my home to work elsewhere. They could not believe the time it had taken me to apply and that despite all the obstacles we had faced with our move, I still wanted to work here! Instantly I felt an ownership and responsibility to these patients that I had never felt in the UK. Here, they truly rely on me. If I am unwell, there is no-one to cover me at work. If I am on holiday, they go without, and again, have to rely on the walk-in centre or emergency room for routine care. I am aware that no-one checks their blood results, investigations or reads their hospital letters if I am away so there is an onus to log on whilst on vacation to keep task lists low and ensure nothing urgent is missed. However, the patients are very respectful of holiday time and encourage me to enjoy my time off, telling me I need the break.

I have more time with my patients in Canada. My appointments are 15 minutes and I see the majority of patients face to face, this was the case even during the third wave of Covid. I offer same day, emergency and phone/virtual appointments. There are not enough GPs in Nova Scotia and the way the system has been set up there is no automatic catchment area for patients. A lot of GPs have more patients than they can manage, so sometimes the wait time for a GP appointment is 6 weeks. The amount of money GPs are remunerated per patient visit is not much, however, the government have recently added enhanced fee codes and different funding for GPs to try to address this. There is no flexible 'part time' option and most doctors work 37.5 hours a week at a minimum. You can work reduced hours but must still be able to offer services for at least 46 weeks across the year, and of course this is reflected in the pay. To be fee for service you have to work hard and see lots of patients. GPs don't want to be overloaded so they get to a certain level and stop taking patients on. Hence more and more people come to the province and have no doctor. Also, there are fewer doctors who want to work in rural areas so the patients there either have no doctor or they have to drive long distances for health care. At the moment the government is concentrating its efforts on recruiting physicians to try to make up the shortfall of family doctors to combat the paucity of GPs across the province.

The question remains: would I ever come back to the NHS, with all its pressures? At the moment, my answer is no. Currently I have 1,200 patients that rely on me, and I don't want to leave them. There are of course problems with the health system and inequalities in Canada, but they exist everywhere and are certainly present in the UK and the NHS. In Canada I feel appreciated and respected. I am happy at work. I have time with my patients. I work hard but my time is flexible. I see more of my children after school and my weekends are free to spend with my family. I am not spending half my weekend catching up on notes and work. My family is settled, and our children are living their best lives here. It is a safer environment for them to grow up in compared to where we lived in the UK. The amenities are not as modern or sophisticated as in the UK, but living is simpler, and the community appreciates the natural beauty surrounding us.

I would not want to go back to the NHS and work in a system where GPs are persistently unappreciated, made the scapegoat for the failing of the government, subject to daily abuse and harassment, and end up burnt out years before retirement. So many of my GP colleagues in the UK are leaving medicine completely due to the stress and pressure they are under. It is unsustainable and I would not want to put my health or my family's livelihood at risk.

I am so pleased to have made the move to Canada, however insidious it was. At the time, I thought that decision was the hardest one we would have to make as a family, but I was wrong: the decision whether to return in the future will ultimately be more difficult.

Health care in Canada

- Health care is free at the point of use to all citizens and permanent residents in Canada.
- The country has a universal publicly funded system called Canadian Medicare. It is funded and administered by each province, which has its own insurance plan.
- Services which are not free include prescriptions, vision and dental care and rehab services.

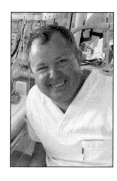

General practice in Norway

Dr Robin Kåss studied medicine in the UK before returning to his homeland of Norway to work as a GP and medical director of the GP-led casualty unit in Skien, Telemark.

In June 2010 he became deputy minister in the Norwegian Ministry of Health. Between 2015–23 he served as mayor of the city of Porsgrunn, alongside his work as an occupational health doctor. He outlines some of the current issues facing general practice in his country, which are only too familiar and mirror those in the UK.

Norway is a country with a population of 5.5 million. The country is wealthy, with a strong welfare state, and consistently ranks as having one of the best healthcare systems in the world.[111]

Secondary health care is organised regionally but owned and funded nationally, while primary health care is the responsibility of the 356 local municipalities. The GP scheme is very popular amongst the inhabitants. However, it has been under increasing strain in the last 10 years. I, myself, used to be a GP, but am now working in both politics and occupational health medicine. I have experienced the scheme as a GP, a politician in national government, mayor in a medium-sized Norwegian city and as family member to users of the service.

Organisational framework

In 2001, the Norwegian government passed a major reform which gave everyone access to a GP. Similar to in the UK, the GP is often the first meeting users have with the health service.[112] Primary health care is organised locally by the municipalities, although the funding and legal framework is national. The number of GPs is not regulated by law or by central authorities; the individual municipality must enter into agreements with GPs to ensure proper health care for its residents.

GPs are responsible for family health clinics and the institutional care of the elderly, and they also take on public health and managing the prison health service, in addition to their normal practice. GPs may also work on call. This varies greatly per region and a rural GP may be on call from home, while a GP in an urban centre will typically be based in a large acute medical centre.

The freedom to organise health care locally is a huge strength in a geographically diverse country like Norway, but also makes the scheme more vulnerable. At times there can be a tendency for the state and local authorities to blame each other for any problems with the system.

Current challenges

Many municipalities are now reporting that it is difficult to recruit GPs. In 2017 the Ministry of Health commissioned a survey to assess the workload for GPs in Norway.[113]

The survey concluded that the average GP workload was 55.6 hours per week (median 52.2). Ten per cent of GPs were working more than 75 hours a week with two thirds of this time spent with patients. There is quite a lot of variation between GPs as to how they use their time, but on average chronically ill patients take 15 per cent, frail elderly 7 per cent and mental health 8 per cent of the time used.

The workload for GPs per patient has increased resulting in the average list size decreasing from 1,200 in 2005 to currently around 1,000. Female GPs have on average less than 1,000 patients. As older GPs retire, and the population increases, this has resulted in a lack of GPs in large parts of Norway. Between 2018 and 2022, the number of GP-lists without a GP has increased from 98 to 310.[114]

The number of vacant patient slots on a GP-list has gone down from 204,594 in 2018 to only 43,386 at the end of 2022. This is a very low number in a country with a population of 5.5 million. People who move can therefore often have difficulties finding a GP in their new area, and this in turn can cause problems for on-call services and for continuity of care.

Everyone residing in a Norwegian municipality has the legal right to have a GP, and the municipality has the duty to provide this service.[115] However the municipalities can't individually address a national shortage of GPs, and a legal right has little value with no available legal remedy for the individual citizen. Municipalities cannot prioritise patients to GPs' lists and the GPs themselves cannot refuse individual patients if they have a vacant slot. New vacant GP slots, as a result of measures by one local authority, may, therefore, often be taken by patients from other municipalities which themselves have a lack of GPs.

Future development

The Norwegian Medical Association has called this a 'GP-crisis',[116] and the new Labour government has appointed a special expert committee to propose solutions.[117] In 2022, the government established a subsidy for municipalities with the greatest recruitment challenges.

This expert committee will investigate how the GP scheme can be made more sustainable. The aims are that overall resources in the health service be used as efficiently as possible, and that the capacity in the GP scheme be increased, for example, by recruiting more doctors, by digitalisation, and by employing other professions to collaborate in GP practices. The committee will also investigate matters related to organisation and funding, including payment rates that facilitate multidisciplinary practices. The committee will propose changes in on-call services so that GPs have reduced working hours in the emergency room and at the same time ensure a good acute service throughout the country. They will also look at possible changes in competence requirements for doctors in the municipal health service.

Hopefully the GP scheme will be strengthened and will remain the jewel and backbone of the Norwegian healthcare system.

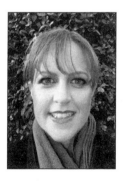

General practice in New Zealand and the UK

Dr Lois Mugleston is a GP working in Nottingham. She was a GP in New Zealand from 2007–15 and owned and ran a practice in semi-rural west Auckland. She reflects on her time there and the initiatives we could take on to dramatically improve the UK experience.

General practice is: 'The point at which the vast undifferentiated mass of human suffering meets the theoretical structures of scientific medicine.'[118]

It is currently an immensely challenging task being a GP in the UK. We have huge issues with workforce. GPs have to deal with a highly stressful and intense job, high workloads and the fallout of the pandemic, with many patients on long waiting lists for surgery or specialist appointments, meaning GPs are looking after them for longer without specialist input, and all the difficulties that entails. Many patients are highly complex, demand is increasing, GP numbers are not increasing, and services are increasingly devolved to the community. It is my experience, in my inner-city Nottingham practice, that the social determinants of health including austerity, poverty, food insecurity, illness, stress levels, poor housing and the significant interpersonal disconnect caused by the pandemic, are increasingly prominent in patients' presentations.

New Zealand

From 2007–15, when I worked as a GP in New Zealand, we rarely saw more than 24 patients in a day. In essence, the workload was less, there were fewer patients per GP, fewer mandatory targets to meet and we had more staff and more time for each patient, with 15-minute appointments as standard. Many salaried GPs had a maximum number of patients per day in their contract; this was a useful benchmark, and most GPs were not expected to routinely exceed this, although we sometimes did on a busy winter's day.

Blood testing was not done by the practice, but by fully funded local phlebotomy services which patients could book their own appointments at, freeing up staff time and phone lines. The practice management system was quick and responsive, with easy inbuilt coding and auditing. There was a much lower administrative burden in terms of letters and documents than there currently is in the UK.

We had time for complex patients, both during appointments and for thinking and administrative time afterwards. We were able to get to know families and their circumstances, so consultations became easier because every patient was not a new patient. Patients never waited more than a day or two for a GP appointment. We were able to refer to hospital specialists in a simple way, with a referral letter rather than having to complete a detailed proforma, and patients were largely seen in a timely manner. There were a few issues with patients waiting quite some time for elective surgery, particularly for general surgery and dermatology. Appointments were able to be expedited if patients deteriorated, but this was sometimes challenging due to a lack of local specialist capacity. We had the ability to close our practice list to new patients once it got too full for the practice to operate safely, helping to prevent an infinite workload and ensuring appropriate access for those registered with us, although to my knowledge we never actually had to do this in any of the four practices I worked at. It was the responsibility of the Ministry of Health to find an alternative GP practice for patients if their local practice had closed its books.[119]

There was an urgent care centre nearby with its own radiology and phlebotomy. It was open on weekends, meaning that some patients with urgent problems went there rather than booking a GP appointment or going to A&E, although we still saw plenty of accidents and did urgent suturing for wounds.

As a result of these largely positive aspects of the job, I usually managed to get home at a reasonable time. Staff were able to take proper lunch breaks and even occasionally go out for lunch. We were able to prioritise time and space for regular team meetings and formulation of an evidence-based strategic plan to deal with the health needs of our local population.

Interesting and practical parts of the job, such as minor surgery, skin biopsy and lesion removal, joint injections, contraceptive device fitting, and palliative care, are retained rather than delegated elsewhere in New Zealand, necessitating a higher skilled GP workforce, but leading to increased job satisfaction.

Patient wellbeing and community

My experience of working in New Zealand was that doctor-patient relationships are valued and preserved, as are relationships between patients and nurses and reception staff, who in my experience were fantastic at facilitating appropriate appointments as well as making patients feel valued and heard. Our reception staff had the time to help patients complete forms if needed, for the few patients in our area who were unable to read, and this helped the staff feel that their roles were valuable and made a difference.

Another key aspect was the general expectations of the population and the culture around health-seeking behaviour. Most patients did not go to see their GP unless they had a medical problem which they could not solve themselves, and many had already been to a pharmacy or tried to treat the problem themselves before seeing the GP. This resulted in a lot less consultation time spent on minor illnesses which typically go away by themselves, such as colds, than we currently see in the UK. Having to pay to see the GP is certainly a good incentive for patients to attempt to self-manage rather than booking an appointment at the first sign of illness, and because this is the norm, many patients also did this with their children despite children's appointments being free.

There were many other services besides general practice to support patients, and these are well-resourced and embedded in local communities, including the community midwife, health visitor, pharmacy, plus a myriad of toddler groups, kids groups at the local library and active groups for seniors. Childcare is exceptionally well funded, with parents only paying a fraction of the actual cost, leading to parents having the ability to choose to work without a large financial barrier if they wished to do so.

At the practice I worked at, patients were grateful for their continuity of care, and the system was set up to support practices and the workforce. Ours was largely a productive and contented workplace; our practice was able to respond to local challenges, listen to staff and adapt our policies to local needs. We had funding for staff training so they could upskill and develop as practitioners. We took part in events such as the village fair, building trust and rapport with the local community.

Public health campaigns in New Zealand are well funded, resourced and coordinated nationwide. This included sun safety, anti-tobacco, anti-alcohol, obesity and diabetes campaigns, as well as anti-gambling measures and speed awareness campaigns. In my opinion, the New Zealand population is far more fit and active than the UK population, aided partly by the weather but also by the normalisation of physical exercise and healthy diet.

Pharmacy and prescription charges

In contrast to the UK, if a medicine is unavailable in New Zealand, pharmacists have the ability to change the prescription to something that is available.[120] The GP is then notified and is able to change the patient's regular prescription if needed. I used to have a short weekly meeting with our local pharmacist about this and we would also be notified ahead of time if things were unavailable locally (which was not very often). This would be an absolute game-changer in the UK because it would save a phenomenal amount of GP and practice staff time, which is currently wasted on phone calls and emails between patients and pharmacists every time a drug, or even a particular strength of a drug, is unavailable. I believe this is something we should consider as a matter of urgency in the UK as it would free up GPs to see more patients.

In New Zealand, patients pay around £2.50 per prescription item at the pharmacy (for subsidised medications), with PHARMAC being the body responsible for deciding what is funded nationally, as well as setting national tariffs and negotiating national discounts.[121] If patients want a particular brand rather than generic, for example Nurofen versus Ibuprofen, or an unsubsidised medication, they need to pay the full cost of this. A prescription subsidy is available once patients have paid for 20 prescription items *per household* in a year, and prescriptions are free for under 14s.[122] In England, current prescription charges are £9.65 per item. Exemptions are available to defined groups, and prescriptions are free for all in Scotland, Wales and Northern Ireland.[123]

General practice funding and registration

Patients are able to register with any GP they like, without any geographical boundary. The downside being that a practice might not be able to take them on if its books were closed. Most patients registered locally for convenience. But, in theory, it is possible to be registered at a practice many miles away if patients wish to do so, as long as they are prepared to travel for their appointments.[124] Patients pay a co-payment of around £20 for their appointment, with the rest government funded. Unregistered patients pay around £35, and international patients around £50. Patients in areas of high socio-economic deprivation pay a lower amount as practices get additional funding. We were allowed to set our fees at whatever level we felt appropriate when we first opened the practice, and after this, annual increases were capped centrally. As a competitive business it did not make sense for us to have a service that was wildly more expensive than surrounding practices.

Children, pregnant women, and those on benefits get free appointments (with the practice appropriately remunerated), as do those with chronic health conditions such as diabetes. Occupational health after accidents are prioritised by use of the no-fault Accident Compensation Corporation (ACC) accident insurance system,[125] meaning patients who have had accidents get free and timely access to tests, specialist appointments, surgery, physiotherapy and workplace-based adaptations, ultimately getting them back to work (and economically productive) soon, rather than languishing on a waiting list for months or years. This system also enables employers with a high incidence of workplace-related accidents to be identified and financially penalised, if necessary, with workplace safety at the fore. Again, in the current economic climate, this is a system the UK could be harnessing, prioritising those off sick from work to get them well again.

I initially found it challenging that patients had to pay for their GP appointment. One senior GP pointed out to me that general practice would not exist in New Zealand if it were not for the co-payments, and that patients would not be able to afford the full cost if they had to pay this, and this helped me to get to grips with it. The co-payment system does help to ensure equity, because those with long-term conditions and on benefits get free appointments. I remember a few patients from the US being surprised at how cheap the appointments were. Patients usually had to pay small additional charges for non-core services such as liquid nitrogen mole removal, ear wax removal and, as a practice, we were able to make a small profit on these to subsidise other parts of the service to ensure we kept patient fees low for general appointments. Patients also had to pay the GP around £5 for repeat prescriptions, meaning that this important work is both recognised and appropriately remunerated. As a managing partner, the patient charges were my responsibility, and it was at my discretion if I decided not to charge a patient for a particular unfunded service. I also occasionally gave patients discounted or free appointments if I felt it was necessary. The co-payments also had the effect of making patients think twice before booking an appointment, as well as encouraging people to self-manage.

There was not the constant mantra of: 'Is that in the contract?' Rather, almost everything was funded appropriately instead of the numerous 'add-ons' to basic contracts and resulting postcode lottery for services that we have in the UK. Extra funding was available for palliative care, the management of depression (longer appointments were fully funded after an appropriate simple and short GP training course), sexual health (free for those aged 16–25) and procedures such as joint injections and ingrowing toenail surgery, as well as for patients who had had accidents. Claiming these costs was quick and simple, the invoicing was integrated into our practice management system and could be done in a few seconds by the GP after each appointment.

There are a few different funding streams, and some funding is target-driven, but nothing compared to the myriad of micro-incentives that GPs are now expected to chase in the UK. The targets that we did have to meet in New Zealand were clear, we had the technological infrastructure to capture the work we had actually done and a clear list of outstanding tasks which we could then easily prioritise. As a result, we were always able to meet our targets each year.

Primary-secondary interface

We had access to patients' hospital records, which helped to improve communication and clarity with what tests had been performed and why. We also had a quick and seamless way of transferring electronic notes instantly when patients moved away, although paper notes still had to be posted. Most people's paper notes were thin volumes, as New Zealand has had electronic patient records for quite some time now. Home visits were virtually unheard of other than for our nursing home and palliative patients. We were also able to decline a home visit if patients lived too far away.

Coming back to the UK

Lois returned to the UK for personal reasons in 2015 and returned to a very different NHS to the one she remembered.

Complexity

The post-pandemic UK health system paints a very different picture from the pre-pandemic one, and there are many lessons we could learn from the systems in New Zealand. Ten-minute appointments are not sufficient to deal with the number and complexity of patients we now see in the UK. Assessing a patient, making a diagnosis and plan, dealing with complex mental health issues, and ensuring patient safety and consistent patient-centred care are virtually impossible to achieve in just 10 minutes. Many specialist referrals are being rejected due to lack of capacity in secondary care, or delayed by requiring a myriad of pre-referral tests, questionnaires and other bureaucratic idiosyncrasies before a referral is accepted. Patients sometimes seek care for emergency medical problems in general practice rather than having to wait a long time in A&E.

Since the Covid-19 pandemic, we now face an unprecedented mental health crisis affecting at least one in six people in Europe. Dr Hans Kluge recently stated at the European Public Health Conference 2022 that: 'We are living in constant crisis mode. We must ensure that we redouble our efforts to prevent illness, promote health, and strengthen day-to-day essential health services.'[126] With ever-increasing demands and responsibilities upon GPs and no additional workforce or funding, it feels as if things are on the verge of collapse. More than half of GPs report suffering abuse from patients.[127] Added to this are 'toxic' media stories about primary care.[128] Sadly, a number of GPs have died by suicide, with no doubt that work pressures are a significant contributing factor.[129]

GP workforce and the healthcare team

In the UK, if a patient lives in the catchment area of a practice, then they can register, regardless of whether the practice has the workforce capacity. In theory, practices can apply to the commissioner to close their lists, but in reality, this poses difficult problems as it has a knock-on impact on surrounding practices, can only be for a maximum of 12 months, and applications may be refused.[130] This does not solve the longer-term problem, that *all* practices are under huge strain.

Shockingly, 474 GP practices have closed permanently between 2013–22.[131] The knock-on effects of closures of nearby practices are keenly felt. Many practices rely on locums to plug gaps, patients often see a different clinician for each appointment, and care is fragmented as a result.

No wonder, then, that many GPs are taking early retirement (contributing to loss of institutional knowledge and wisdom passed on to younger colleagues), and two thirds of GP trainees plan to work part time once they qualify.[132] In my practice, two senior partners have retired early in the past 12 months, with another set to retire in the next 6 months. Training places have historically remained unfilled[133] and now as many as one in six qualified GP positions are vacant.[134] Many GPs are suffering burnout, and there is good evidence that patient safety declines as a result of this, with burnt-out GPs twice as likely to be involved in a safety incident.[135]

All primary care staff – doctors, nurses, reception, administrative, healthcare assistants, physician assistants (PAs), pharmacists, social prescribers, IT support – are a vital part of well-functioning health care. In my recent salaried position, two senior partners have retired early in the past 12 months, with another set to retire in the next 6 months. The practice has a very experienced advanced nurse practitioner (ANP) due to retire in the next 6 months, and no-one to replace her. This will invariably have a huge impact on workload. All GPs interface with many other community-orientated services including the palliative care team, district nurses, midwives, health visitors, social workers, school nurses, the mental health team, community pharmacists, dieticians, podiatrists, opticians, dentists, community alcohol and drug teams, community respiratory and cardiac teams and many others, all of whom are also under strain.

Workload

The BMA report 'Safe Working in General Practice' recommends 25 patient contacts per day in order for a GP to deliver safe care.[136] Horrifyingly, a recent poll suggested that GPs are delivering 84 per cent more contacts than the safe limit.[137]

The RCGP has projected that general practice will lose around 18,950 GPs and trainees over the next 5 years unless steps are taken to tackle intense workload and workforce pressures.[138] There are many ways that this could be achieved. However, currently many GPs are simply firefighting, struggling to stay on top of the immense workload, meaning that higher level strategising is simply not able to occur.

Patient demand has been rising even prior to the pandemic,[139, 140] for multiple reasons. We now have large numbers of patients waiting for specialist appointments, who are being managed by GPs in the interim. We also find that patients seek GP help when other services could be more appropriately utilised instead, such as self-managing for self-limiting conditions, things a pharmacist could deal with, or for problems that require attendance at A&E. In many cases the only support for mental health are charitable organisations that can be limited in scope, or a few sessions on the NHS, which is insufficient for treating even the most basic of issues. Schemes such as the Sure Start programme for children and families had been shown to prevent 13,150 hospital admissions annually, but these are now being defunded, with 500 sites already closed.[141, 142]

Many sectors now indemnify themselves with the request for people to 'consult your GP', or 'get a letter from your GP', as if somehow a GP's seal of approval is required for every self-help action. The constant need for 'access' has not been balanced by an equal and opposing force, and I would say patients should not have access to a GP at all costs, rather, *appropriate* access is what is required, i.e. when people actually *need* a GP, as opposed to self-managing, or consulting another service.

Bureaucracy of returning

The simple act of returning to work in the UK as a GP from New Zealand has been hugely challenging, even though I attained my medical degree in the UK. Despite being a highly competitive and high-level training course, New Zealand GP qualifications are not automatically recognised in the UK. Because I completed my GP training there, this meant I had to undertake the arduous process of obtaining the

Certificate of Eligibility for GP Registration (CEGPR), a process that is so stringent and bureaucratic, that fewer than five GPs worldwide manage to get through each year, with some years the rejection rate being 100 per cent.[143]

Requirements to work as a UK GP

To be able to work as an independent, unsupervised GP in the UK, doctors are required to:

- Be on the GMC GP register and hold a GMC licence to practice.
- Be on the national performers' list.

Getting onto the GP register requires completion of a medical degree (5–6 years) and then completion of foundation and GP training (5 years). For overseas doctors, the process is even more complicated. Experienced GPs who did not train in the UK, or doctors, such as Lois, who have worked outside of the UK for 2 years, must tick a series of expensive and time-consuming boxes before they can join or re-join the NHS workforce. Overseas doctors must first obtain the CEGPR, a process that can take up to a year in collecting paperwork and providing evidence. All doctors must then undergo a process called the GP Induction and Refresher Scheme (I&R Scheme).[144]

Despite 6 months of careful planning and preparation prior to leaving New Zealand, it still took a further 18 months to get on the GP register, the performers' list and complete the requirements of the scheme. I believe that the process has been somewhat truncated now, but it still remains a huge barrier for overseas GPs coming to work in the UK. The 'training' provided in the I&R Scheme was in fact working as a GP with the odd tutorial and a bit of study time thrown in. I was fortunate to have a supportive practice, but the whole process was still incredibly lengthy and stressful. I believe it is imperative to remove these bureaucratic barriers if we are to meet the needs of our population.

Moving forward

It is a political choice to underfund primary care and public health in the NHS, and to fail to improve staff numbers and working conditions despite the stresses of the pandemic. These issues have been going on for years but have been accelerated by the pandemic. Many European countries have more GPs per head of population and spend more per head than we do in the UK.[145] It is vital that we invest in primary care and public health preventative strategies.

As a GP who has previously suffered from burnout, a sustainable career is a must. For me, this means working in a range of varied roles, including at a local nursing home, teaching trainees and medical students, doing GP appraisals and working in the medicines optimisation team, alongside patient-facing work as well as remote sessions. Many GPs now have this portfolio-style career. Patient-facing roles have become intense and bogged down with endless admin. If we can achieve better in-practice variety and depth, perhaps more GPs will be able to increase their clinical workload.

A colleague has solved workforce issues at her practice by employing a number of PAs to help process the simpler parts of the job. Training took time, which not every practice would be able to offer, but they have now become an integral part of their team. GPs need to have the mental space to think deeply about their patients' needs, to ultimately improve patient satisfaction, safety and outcomes. Home visits can take a large chunk of GPs' time (up to 1 hour per visit). Other members of the multidisciplinary team, such as paramedics and advanced nurse practitioners, have the skills to do these visits with support. We also need to take care not to overburden GP trainees with our own excessive workloads, lest they burn out and leave before they have really begun their careers.

Appointments for complexity

Patients don't always *need* to see a GP, and many conditions can be safely self-managed or managed by other services. In parallel to this, transitioning to 15-minute GP appointments would enable complex patients to be properly dealt with. It is vital that GPs have access to adequate support for the increasing numbers of patients with mental health problems and patients in poverty. Long term, the social determinants of health need to be addressed, as these account for up to 55 per cent of health outcomes.[146] Reducing health inequalities goes hand in hand with this, and without a fully funded and fully resourced NHS we risk exacerbating inequality.

GP funding

To prevent general practice going the disastrous way of NHS dentistry, it is imperative that appropriate funding is urgently put into place. We need finances for safe and appropriate staffing levels, the ability to train PAs and other patient support roles, fixing crumbling buildings, and to ensure we have a sustainable workforce and safe workload whilst patients are able to access primary care in appropriate ways. Adding funding complexity and more micro-incentives will not help and is only likely to make more people retire early.

Health promotion and prevention

There have been huge cuts to public health funding in the UK, with a reduction of 24 per cent, or £1 billion in real terms since 2015.[147] As a result, our nation has become sicker, and we are storing up problems for years to come. Prevention of ill health is key to a health system that functions well, and there is good evidence for this.[148, 149] The NHS is drowning in work caused by preventable or partly preventable illnesses and would undoubtedly be less overloaded if more prevention strategies were in place, and healthy lifestyles at the forefront of our government's policies, as is the case in New Zealand.

Staff wellbeing

I have recently taken the 'life values inventory' questionnaire.[150] For me, it's been really revealing about why working in general practice has become so challenging. My number one important value came out as 'belonging'. I imagine that it's something important for many people, and it's one of the reasons why I enjoy working as part of a team so much, because of the sense of belonging and purpose it creates, reducing professional isolation, sharing the burden of complex and difficult patients, supporting each other and being able to bounce ideas off each other, leading to better ideas, innovative solutions to problems, and a sense of perspective.

Since the pandemic, this has been hugely eroded, with staff eating lunch alone at desks while slogging through the workload, or in the car between visits, meaning colleagues don't see each other.[151] This is unhealthy and unsustainable long term. Regular team meetings improve communication, teamwork, and identify issues and their solutions more readily. With such huge workload pressures, making time for team meetings has understandably not been prioritised.

It is imperative that GPs have the mental space for higher level systems thinking, as well as time for connecting with colleagues,[152] caring for each other, and for basic human needs such as going to the toilet, eating lunch, getting out of the chair to stretch and giving overworked brains a rest so we can think clearly and optimally rather than each day being 'adrenaline-soaked survival'.[153] Simple changes will enable GPs to have sustainable careers, stay in the workforce for longer, reduce clinician suicide rates, and ultimately will benefit patient safety.

Appointment bookings

My practice has responded to the increasing workload and high patient non-attendance rates by adding more on-the-day appointments and reducing pre-booked appointments. This is good for dealing with acute demand, but also impacts patients by reducing ability to book appointments in advance, making things more difficult for those with chronic conditions as well as patients who work or care for others, who may not have the ability to stay on the phone for prolonged periods of time waiting to get through, or to have an appointment the same day without prearranging with their employer or childcare. It is impossible to find a system that works for everyone.

Flexible working

As technology improves, remote work as a GP is becoming easier, with a number of private recruitment firms now advertising remote-only jobs. If the NHS could harness the GPs applying for these jobs rather than haemorrhaging staff to private companies with better working conditions, this would go some way to improving the workforce crisis, making it more attractive to continue to work as a GP for those with young children, or those nearing retirement. Some GPs may have the ability to do part sessions remotely rather than whole sessions, contributing to the overall number of appointments available whilst working sustainably.

Right clinician/right time

There are many tasks I perform in the working day which could be done by other practitioners, and this was also found to be the case in the King's Fund Report.[154] Sharing out workload across skilled practitioners whilst reserving GPs to do 'only things a GP can do' seems sensible. The practicalities of this may be challenging, as we are dealing with undifferentiated illness presentations, which can often be vague. Not all patients need to be seen immediately, and many patients with chronic conditions or routine appointments can safely wait a few weeks. Accurate triage is clearly important.

Improving workflow

Optimal time management is also important. Being interrupted causes significant disruptions to thought processes, especially if the interruption is not related to the current task,[155, 156] so I'd like to outlaw instant messaging and instead communicate through tasks or emails that I check when I am available, unless it is a medical emergency. My practice does not have an electronic patient-calling system, meaning that minutes of that precious appointment time are wasted walking to and from the waiting room.

During telephone clinics, I frequently experience wrong numbers and have to call patients back later, which wastes time and effort. We are already using text messaging, phone and video calling to optimise communication, and much more that could be done in this area. Automating processes would help (for example, sending patients electronic information leaflets). We must be careful not to overload patients with marginal or irrelevant communications, and we must continue having discussions about very important topics directly with patients, although this could be done by telephone or video call.

Reducing the bureaucracy of hospital acute and outpatient referral systems will be beneficial, although many practices employ secretaries to take some of the burden of this now, anything that helps GPs stick to the core business of being a GP will help. Some areas still require the GP to phone the on-call registrar to refer patients in acutely. Personally, I think this is a waste of everyone's time. I have worked in a hospital where GP referrals were sent straight to A&E and seen directly by the relevant team (medicine, surgery, etc.) and largely this worked well. Phone calls to hospital colleagues could be reserved for when the GP needs advice about keeping the patient in the community rather than a patient who obviously needs admission.

Finally, protected time and funding for GP learning not only improves patient experiences and safety but is also vital to cultivating an engaged and curious workforce who will be able to sustain enjoyable careers until retirement. This will help prevent the early exodus of some, and

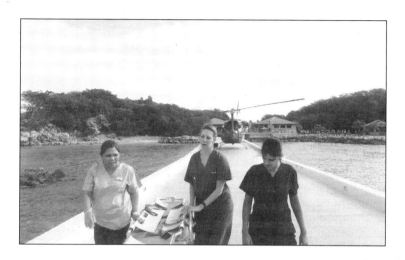

will benefit patients by having happy and interested GPs who enjoy what they do, as well as improving knowledge, communication and patient safety. The future, as I currently see it, is fragile.

The American system – fees at sea

Do patients get better care outside of the UK? One of the solutions often raised to solve the problems within primary care is to attach a price tag and create an American-style system where there are upfront charges for care. Across the pond, healthcare costs are the number one cause of bankruptcy for Americans and 56 million people struggle with medical debt each year.[157] I experienced working within an 'American-style' system during my time as a cruise ship doctor, and I explain here why I don't think we should adopt this approach within the NHS. A version of the piece below first appeared in metro.co.uk in January 2023 and is reproduced here with permission.[158]

I spent many years working as a cruise ship doctor. I travelled the world dealing with quite a lot more than a spot of sea sickness. People get unwell at sea in the same way they do on land: from coughs, colds, dislocations and stitches, to heart attacks, strokes, and critically ill patients needing intensive care level support. The main thing I learnt from all this, was just how important travel insurance is. A cruise can be idyllic, until you get ill. To the dismay of many British guests, medical care on cruise ships comes with a hefty bill.

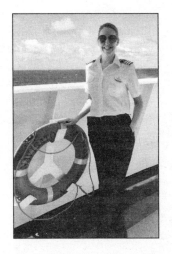

This is why I fiercely oppose former UK Health Secretary Sajid Javid's proposal[159] to introduce fees for GP appointments and A&E visits. His idea isn't new. Debates over NHS fees have raged since the creation of the service, and the evidence[160] we have for charging patients shows time and time again that even with exemptions in place, a fee to see the doctor widens health inequalities by deterring the poor and vulnerable from seeking help.

I recall the elderly lady who shuffled to the nurse's station onboard the ship looking fairly well. She asked about the consultation fees, then decided against a visit. Twenty-four hours later, the whole medical team was summoned over the Tannoy to her cabin, to find her in extremis, from a condition that could have been prevented had we only seen her earlier.

Another patient needed to be medically disembarked from the ship with an acute abdomen for surgical care on land. The ambulance was waiting on the pier to transport her to hospital, but the patient flatly refused to get on board. We were in the US, and being American herself, she knew there was a fee for ambulance transport which her insurance didn't cover. She took an Uber instead (and subsequently needed to have surgery for her problem).

On another cruise, a patient without medical insurance was having a heart attack. Miles from land, in a critical condition she needed to have a clot busting treatment. The decision had been made to administer this potentially life-saving medication, but just as we opened the cupboard to draw it up, the chief nurse took me aside and whispered to me, 'Docky, have you asked their partner if they're happy to pay for this?' It cost $7,000 a vial. I then had to go and have *that* conversation with an already incredibly stressed relative.

A cruise ship is a microcosm of society, and all these examples will play out on a wider scale if fees are introduced to the NHS. The unintended consequences will far outweigh the financial gains, which will need to be offset by the huge costs in policing and administering a payment system.

A recurring argument in favour of charging in the UK is the one that presumes a fee will reduce the 'unnecessary' presentations. The patients that 'don't need to be there'. 'If people have to pay a fee to see their GP, then they will think twice about presenting.' Well, I would disagree. I remember many patients happily paying at least $100 to see me on board the ship, when their money would be better spent elsewhere: the lad in his twenties worried about a black mark on his fingernail which turned out to be dirt under his nail which I removed for him (for no extra charge). For me it may have seemed unnecessary, but who is the judge of that? If he felt reassured that the black spot wasn't cancer, then to him it was money well spent.

But the fact that a fee is in place does raise ethical questions. If a doctor asks for a follow-up visit, are they being caring or will they be branded money-making? We all heard rumours on ships about the early days of cruise ship medicine, where staff worked on commission: stories of patients attending with a cold, and being offered X-rays, swabs and bloods, and a host of expensive treatments, all for a substantial bill. As paying customers, patients may want the reassurance of a barrage of tests – unnecessary tests can have harm attached – assigning a fee to health care changes the dynamic completely.

Javid advocated introducing these fees, to 'help with the allocation of limited resources'. 'What frustrates people,' said Javid, 'is having to wait for GP appointments.'[161] When I had a busy clinic on board, and a waiting room full of sick, paying passengers, they still all had to wait to see me. A consultation fee doesn't help with waiting times. Just look at the waits for NHS dentistry if you're not convinced.

Chapter 6
The future of general practice

There is genuine discontent within primary care right now, both from patients, trying to get their problems heard, and the professionals working within a failing system. If you've made it this far through the book, then you have heard many of the reasons for our predicament, and many potential solutions have already been raised.

The increased demands of the pandemic did have a silver lining, in that they showed just how innovative primary care teams can be. The pandemic response in setting up hot hubs, shifting to remote working, safeguarding care homes, and, later, delivering the vaccination programme, was lifesaving, and done rapidly at short notice. Things may be bleak within the NHS, but what continues to give hope is the willingness of people to work together to find solutions.

Many of the bigger solutions, such as funding, infrastructure and social care reform, need to come from our NHS leaders, but there are many smaller-scale solutions which can be developed locally within our communities. There are also changes we can make as individuals – both as patients using the service and as professionals – things we can do ourselves and demands we can make of the system to try to improve things.

This chapter looks towards solutions. First, a GP, who wishes to remain anonymous, examines the role of allied health care professionals (AHCPs) and looks at working at scale within primary care networks (PCNs). Then I discuss part-time GPs and take a closer look at how working time is defined within general practice, and how a rebrand is needed to simply illustrate the unseen workload within GP teams. This has been described as the 'part-time paradox'. If the public consensus is that GPs are lazy slackers, while the daily reality is a relentless slog, there's a total disconnect, and the problems are less likely to be solved until we move onto the same page.

I want to return to the book I mentioned earlier, *A Fortunate Woman*, which describes how the 'accumulated knowledge' of a family doctor helped the GP to really 'see' her patients, and know them as people within their communities, rather than as their illnesses. One of the mechanisms linking continuity of care to better outcomes for patients is this 'accumulated knowledge', which is essentially a relationship – getting to know someone over many years. You get to know them, their families and their struggles. When I worked as a GP in the Lake District, I hadn't been around long enough to acquire this skill, but I recall valuing it highly in the reception team, who had worked there for years, also living in the village with everyone on our patient list. They could take one look at someone sitting in the waiting room and know things weren't quite right. They knew the stories and the relationships, and that information is sometimes much more useful than a blood pressure and a pulse rate. Being the crew doctor on cruise ships was similar – I lived and worked with these people, knew the pressures of their job and the personalities in their lives.

Continuity of care has steadily declined over the last decade. The *British Journal of General Practice* showed that between 2012–17 the percentage of patients able to see their preferred GP fell by 10 percentage points. Not everyone wants that continuity it seems, as the percentage of patients who reported having a preferred GP also fell by nine percentage points.[162] People seem to want different things at different stages of life, and transactional medicine is exactly what some people want. But when illness takes hold, and visits to hospital and doctors surgeries become more frequent than we would like, having someone there who knows us, who we have a relationship with, is worth its weight in gold. I miss that as a remote doctor, and my fondest 'work memories' are the ones involving those relationships – it works both ways.

The book finishes with a summary of potential solutions. Then, it's over to you, the reader, to think about how as users of the service, we can all safely get the most out of it. The thing about being a GP, is that we know very well that one day we are going to be a patient on the other side too, and making the system better is in all of our interests.

Are allied healthcare professionals a solution to the GP crisis?

Despite general practice being one of the few areas of the NHS where productivity is higher than before the pandemic, with consultation figures at a record high, patients continue to report problems in booking appointments with GPs. We know that the number of qualified GPs working in the

NHS has fallen in recent years, despite government pledges to substantially increase numbers. An anonymous GP explores the role of non-GPs in the future of NHS general practice.

The UK has fewer hospital beds than most comparable countries
Total hospital beds per 1,000 inhabitants

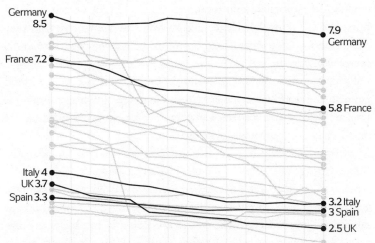

Safe staffing levels are critical to the running of any healthcare system. We know that the UK has one of the lowest numbers of hospital beds and doctors per head of population of all the OECD nations.[163] (See above and also the graph on page 91 of Chapter 5.)

The lack of a credible workforce plan is an ongoing concern for all healthcare professionals, and one of the reasons many doctors have (overwhelmingly and often reluctantly) voted to strike. For many doctors the industrial action is not about 'pay'; it is about creating a culture and working environment that will support and retain staff, in modern functional healthcare facilities which will allow the NHS to provide safe, efficient care.

You have seen throughout this book how the wider NHS, and more specifically, general practice, is struggling to meet patient demand. The data shows that around 90 per cent of all NHS contacts occur in general practice, yet the budget allocated to it represents around 8 per cent of NHS spending.[164] Data also shows that we have a growing population (in size as well as numbers), living with ever more complex medical conditions which require more care and support from GP teams. In addition to managing long-term conditions, GPs are also expected to offer urgent access for minor illness and emergencies, along with health screening and vaccination programmes. Demand for appointments has been steadily growing, yet there are fewer GPs working, due to a variety of reasons such as burnout, early retirement, emigration, less than full time training (LTFT) working and the pursuit of a 'portfolio' career. Many GPs choose to assist hospital clinics or work in urgent care centres, out-of-hours providers, and, increasingly, in the private sector.

To compound matters, demand is much higher now than pre-pandemic. Practices are merging into larger groups, hospital waiting lists are at record levels (meaning more patients are contacting GP practices for support while waiting) and there are fewer GP partners. Assuming the stats continue, there will soon be a majority of 'salaried' (non-partner) GPs. This is in fact a stated aim of the current Labour party, who, at the time of writing, are looking likely to win the next general election (currently theirs to lose). Nobody knows how a salaried GP workforce would deliver services, and the NHS has only even known a partner-led GP model. Most health experts (and anyone working in general practice) recognise that GP partners carry a huge unpaid burden in terms of practice management, organising quality outcomes, compliance, regulation, HR, estates management, training, mentoring and leadership. The idea of GP practices eventually being run by corporate chains would be a seismic shift from the 'ye olde family GP' that many of us 'grew up with', and personally fills me with concern.

Despite increasing the numbers of GP trainees,[165] there is a very high attrition rate, and the number of full time equivalent (FTE) qualified GPs working in the NHS has fallen, despite government pledges to substantially increase (for more figures, see Chapter 4 'What does a GP do in today's Britain?'). Covid forced the entire NHS to 'go digital', resulting in a sea change in the way people access and book with their GP practice, and the whole system lurched into an emergency 'on the day footing'. In many ways, nationally we are still to find a healthy balance post-Covid between 'on-the-day access' versus 'long-term conditions' care.

This toxic combination is a perfect storm for the 'GP crisis', and explains why patients are struggling to see a GP, why patients now struggle to have a regular GP (continuity of care) and explains why the national annual GP surveys[166] understandably show a steady decline in access, satisfaction and continuity.

Solutions to the GP crisis

Strong and accessible primary care services are the foundations of an effective healthcare system.[167] Research shows that the ratio of primary care physicians to population is directly related to health outcomes.[168] Turnover of GP staff affects quality of care, and is worse in deprived areas, further exacerbating health inequalities.[169] There is also strong evidence that continuity of care reduces morbidity, increases life expectancy[170] and improves satisfaction for patients and healthcare professionals.

Whilst think tanks and policy makers are suggesting new ways of working, many GPs are reducing their hours, retiring early or emigrating. In the last few years, despite a lack of evidence, NHS policy has been to encourage GPs to work at scale, for example, in PCNs, with increasing reliance on AHCPs to support a dwindling medical workforce.[171]

The recent push began in January 2019 with a scheme to expand the role of pharmacists within general practice.[172] At the time there was an excess of pharmacists in the community, highly skilled in pharma but also offering 'over the counter' remedies, immunisations and advice on minor injuries and illness. In 2019, there were very few pharmacists working within GP teams. Utilising their obvious expertise in medicine management and their ability (with training and supervision in general practice) to deal with both acute and long-term conditions has been a huge success. Today, pharmacists are a core part of most practice teams and they are indispensable (no pun intended). Anecdotally, it is becoming harder to recruit into community pharmacy, but this is the story for every profession if 'poached' into GP practices. Pharmacists are now embedded in many general practices, offering medication reviews, helping manage long-term conditions and overseeing medicine management.

In early 2023, health secretary Steve Barclay, announced plans to further expand the role of medical support staff in the NHS to relieve pressure on GPs, aiming to improve access to services.[173] This included provision for the GMC to regulate physician associates (PAs) for the first time.

A PA will hold a science degree, and then undergo 2 years of postgraduate clinical training with mentoring. PAs have worked in the US since the 1960s, but were only introduced in the UK in 2003, initially in hospitals.

Since the PCN Additional Roles Reimbursement Scheme (ARRS) granted funding for PAs in April 2022, the PA role has expanded in primary care in England. They are also being increasingly used to boost the Welsh workforce.[174] In the UK, PAs will eventually be GMC registered.[175] Once approved by the GMC, and when trained and competent, PAs would be able to carry out many of the duties of a medically trained doctor. This could include diagnosing illnesses, performing diagnostic and therapeutic procedures, and developing treatment management plans. The potential advantages are clear: a large NHS workforce with more rapid training than doctors, on a lower pay scale, who have the potential to support medical teams in their work, and to improve access to primary care services.

These changes have been met with much debate within the profession. *British Medical Journal* columnist and GP, Helen Salisbury, raised concerns about the dilution of skills these roles bring, unconvinced they reduce workload: 'You need expertise on the frontline. With lots of these first contact roles you increase activity but not necessarily efficiency. When I'm feeling pessimistic, I worry the use of roles like PAs are a deliberate attempt to downgrade general practice.'[176]

In the summer of 2023, two news stories caught my eye. Firstly, on 12 June 2023 the first TAVI (keyhole valve replacement) procedure was fully completed by an 'advanced nurse practitioner' resulting in a social media storm.[177]

The hospital proclaimed this a 'true transformation addressing NHS needs' while many cardiologists expressed concerns about patient safety and removing training for junior doctors. Secondly, around the same time, news broke about a PA working at a GP practice where a patient died after the PA failed to diagnose a deep vein thrombosis (DVT) – a blood clot in the leg. The patient, Emily Chesterton, saw the same PA twice with breathlessness and calf pain and believed they were seeing a doctor. She was misdiagnosed with a sprain, long covid and anxiety. A coroner concluded she was likely to have survived if referred for emergency care at either appointment.[178]

This story also provoked a heated and furious debate in both the medical and national press about the pros and cons of AHCPs.

In October 2023, over 2800 doctors signed a letter written by the Doctors' Association urging the GMC to reconsider plans to regulate PAs, describing them as unsafe and premature.[179] In November, the

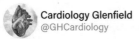

Cardiology Glenfield
@GHCardiology

Momentous day for Glenfield, UHL and the whole world. John is the first nurse-ANP who has performed the whole TAVI procedure as the first operator 👍 true transformation addressing NHS needs. Congratulations John we are so proud of you 🙌 @UHLRRCV @RMitchell_NHS @Leic_hospital

---

A TAVI is a transcatheter aortic valve implantation that improves blood flow to the heart by replacing a damaged aortic valve. Cardiologists took to X (formerly Twitter) raising patient safely concerns, stating that being an operator is about much more than just the procedure and patients need a clinician who can manage their complexities pre and post procedure as well. Doctors currently struggle to obtain opportunities to carry out such procedures, and this is another example of how our trainee doctors are being deskilled as their training is given to the very clinicians who will turn to them for advice in the future.

BMA called for an immediate halt to the recruitment of medical associate professionals until the government and NHS put guarantees in place to ensure proper regulation and supervision.[180]

Dr Matt Kneale, co-chair of DAUK said; 'The rapid expansion of PAs in the NHS threatens to undermine patient safety and the foundations of general practice. While PAs can provide some support, they lack the comprehensive training and expertise of GPs. Relying on PAs as a shortcut solution risks misdiagnoses and inappropriate referrals, as tragically evidenced by recent cases. We cannot allow the role of highly qualified GPs to be diluted and downgraded. The focus must remain on urgently addressing the root causes of workforce shortages, not hastily creating a two-tier system that puts patients at risk.'

How can PAs integrate safely?

As it is a relatively new role, the work of a PA is sometimes not clearly understood. The best analogy is midwives. We all recognise the skill and expertise of midwives (who are not doctors), yet they are rightly recognised as experts in pregnancy care and delivery. The same is true for clinical nurse specialists (CNS), who are widely depended upon in many areas of the NHS.

PAs already give this same level of support in many specialties across the US. Though not expected to manage the more complicated, and sometimes life-threatening, situations for which we rely on doctors, PAs could safely take workload pressures off other members of the primary care team.

Apart from direct patient care, including home visits, in primary care, PAs can be trained in specific disease areas (for example frailty, respiratory disease or diabetes) and can gain skills including joint injections and minor surgery. With support and training, PAs could also help with much of the day-to-day administrative work, such as managing pathology results, ensuring clinical targets are met, and dealing with incoming clinical correspondence.

We know GPs are in short supply, and despite political promises, numbers are still falling. Medical schools in the UK graduate around 9,500 students annually. According to the Medical Schools Council, this needs to be increased to 14,500 new graduates a year. And that's just the beginning of training. After medical school, there are a minimum of 5 additional years of postgraduate training before a doctor is fully licensed to practise independently as a GP, so we need better solutions.

Although PAs can help, we do not yet have enough of them. In 2020, there were about 36,000 active GPs in England[181] and there are approximately 2,850 PAs.[182] In the US there are currently 576,693 primary care physicians[183] and 132,940 PAs.[184] That's one PA supporting 12 doctors in the UK compared with one PA supporting four in the US. This is further complicated when you consider that only a proportion of UK PAs are currently based in general practice.[185]

With any healthcare professional, the person and their competence, rather than their job title, are key. With the high complexity and variety which presents in general practice, dealing with undifferentiated symptoms, any AHCPs joining a GP team will need intensive ongoing training and support for many months (perhaps years) to help them become competent and mitigate risk.

At present, there are no standards for this, and little, if any, protected time or funding for training and supervision. With increasing reliance on support staff, many GPs do not appreciate how much of their own time they will need to invest in training and supervising AHCPs. Guidance on these roles has been minimal.

Working at scale –
primary care networks (PCNs)

Apart from bringing AHCPs into GP, the other main policy focus has been 'working at scale'.

In January 2019, GP practices in England were asked to form primary care networks (PCNs) to serve 30,000–50,000 patients within shared geographical areas. Asking practices to work together at scale was a key policy of the 2019 NHS Long Term Plan.[186] Whilst not obliged to join a PCN, practices were heavily incentivised by the additional funding available. Deadlines were short. Larger practices were able to form a PCN alone, but the vast majority of practices had to rapidly join up with others. Since July 2019, PCNs have increasingly become the focus for primary care development and investment, with new initiatives, such as the Investment and Impact Fund (IIF), being organised and distributed through the networks.

Working at scale facilitates offering population-based health services, employing a wider range of clinical staff and expertise to improve patient care. Patients prefer to be seen closer to home, and care is often more efficient in primary care, so developing community-level services and preventing onward referral to hospitals is both cost-effective and popular. The rationale behind potential improvement in patient care from collaboration is based on economies of scale. Collaboration including sharing best practices, integrating IT systems and exchange of information facilitates a learning environment and results in gained efficiencies. Positive impacts of large-scale practice collaborations, however, depend on their structure and implementation.

The main advantage of PCNs is having funding for extra staff. Given the well-recognised 'GP crisis', central policy has been funding for AHCPs. AHCPs provide specialised services, freeing up GPs' time and easing demands on primary care. The range of staff that can be employed is dictated by the ARRS, with most PCNs employing practice-based pharmacists, social prescribers, paramedics, physios, PAs and mental health workers. Dieticians and occupational therapists can also be employed, but they do not seem to be popular. In addition to the ARRS, money has been allocated for development and education and towards a clinical director.

There are inflexibilities in the ARRS, such as restrictions on types of staff recruited, and the inability to roll over unspent budget into following years or spend it on anything apart from staff. This can be particularly challenging where budgets are devolved within PCNs in proportion to the list sizes of constituent practices. Sharing staff can raise issues with allocating workload, using multiple IT systems or understanding varying protocols. Like any new enterprise, legal agreements are required, funded by the practices, with much discussion about structures and voting rights. PCNs can become another layer of bureaucracy requiring regular meetings with associated preparation time and increased email traffic.

Working in groups and sharing staff can bring tensions. Many PCNs have seen clinical directors change, and practices come and go due to disputes. New staff require recruitment, training and supervision, which is not accounted for, and is especially challenging with remote working. Integrating into large teams can be difficult for staff, especially if working across multiple sites. Training reception staff to understand ARRS staff roles and to appropriately signpost patients takes time. Some patients prefer to see 'their' GP over AHCPs, and larger teams risk eroding continuity of care. Finding desk space and clinical rooms for expanding teams poses another major problem, with many practices already struggling to accommodate existing staff.

As for other organisational models of general practice, like super-partnerships and federations, research and evidence in this area is scarce. In 2021, there were around 1,250 PCNs across England. Since their establishment, GPs' discontentment with the accompanying GP contract that was implemented has been well-documented. However, an early evaluation indicated an overall positive effect on services provision,[187] at least from an operational standpoint. PCNs were integrated rapidly, including swift recruitment of staff into ARRS roles and establishment of enhanced patient services. However, how this translates to health outcomes or quality of care is uncertain. No conclusive qualitative or quantitative evidence on the topic exists to date.

Despite a lack of evidence on the impact of PCNs on patient outcomes, several learning points have emerged. Firstly, PCNs provide a nationally aligned framework for co-working between GP practices. Whilst the consistency of resulting outcomes is to be determined, this has resulted in a clearer direction for practices expanding their services at the community level. Secondly, this framework is not overly prescriptive and does not prevent practices from having autonomy. Even in terms of operational aspects of PCNs, there is significant variety. For example, whilst initially devised as networks covering a population of 30,000–50,000 patients, in practice a lot of the established networks are either smaller or (more often) larger than this.

The Covid-19 pandemic presented opportunities for PCNs to deliver population-based care at scale. Many PCNs spearheaded the vaccination rollout, with GP teams providing around 75 per cent of vaccines. Social prescribers made an impact in supporting shielding patients, and continue to support vulnerable and frail patients in the community. PCNs have developed home visiting and minor illness teams, first contact physios, mental health teams and pharmacy teams to ease GPs' workload. Future opportunities may include further vaccine rollouts, tackling health inequalities, introducing long-Covid clinics, providing community specialist services and improved cancer diagnosis. One challenge will be seizing these opportunities whilst operating within a changing NHS landscape and PCNs establishing their role as a 'building block' of the newer integrated care systems (ICS).

Change is coming

Change is coming. We can see this from the Policy Exchange White Paper[188] and Fuller Report.[189] With consistent failure to deliver repeated promises to boost GP numbers, it is clear that we will be increasingly relying on AHCPs, including PAs, in the future. As such, we need clear standards around training and supervision, a clear regulatory structure along with robust qualitative and quantitative data for outcomes from allied health professionals. We also need the public to understand the benefits of non-GP clinical staff in primary care, and for policy makers to plan how this care can be provided safely.

PAs offer one solution to the workforce crisis in general practice, but they will need considerable support from other members of the primary care team. Careful evaluation of the PA role in primary care is also needed to ensure this is a clinically effective and cost-effective intervention which does not have negative impacts on NHS costs, patient safety, quality of care and health outcomes.

There is clear potential for PCNs to provide population-based health care at scale, improve patient services, bring extra AHCPs into general practice and reduce existing pressures on GPs. It would be good to see evolving evidence emerge regarding the benefits and opportunities for

PCNs, and I would urge the government to scrutinise healthcare policy in the same way as we scrutinise new medicines or treatments before rolling them out.

In my own view – having worked in the NHS for many years – it is always the amazing, dedicated staff who are the glue holding the system together. As one of my close friends says: 'I'm just a tiny cog in a huge dysfunctional system.' This is all too true, and I think we have to take a step back and ask ourselves: 'What makes a good healthcare professional?' (Let's leave the 'allied' out of it for now, because it's almost derogatory.)

For me, it's all about the Cs. And if we strive for these qualities across all roles within our healthcare system, the patients will not mind if they see a consultant, trainee nurse, paramedic, GP or healthcare assistant, so long as they get the right care in the right place by the right person in the right manner.

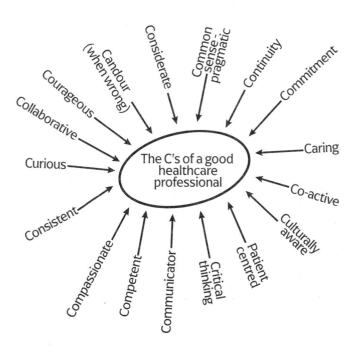

Are part-time GPs the problem?

GPs are well overdue a rebrand when it comes to how working hours are defined. This alone may open the eyes of commentors who talk disparagingly about 'part-time' GPs with a roll of the eyes. I highlight just what 'part time' means in general practice and how understanding and embracing part timers, rather than vilifying them may offer another solution to our GP workforce crisis. A version of the following piece first appeared on metro. co.uk and is reproduced here with permission.[190]

'Why do so many GPs work part time these days?' asked a patient at the end of a consultation. I found myself blustering through a reply about workload, clinical pressures and decision-making fatigue. A few weeks later, another part-time GP friend tells me she was asked the same thing. 'I'm deeply offended by that question,' she replied. I realised that I had been too.

According to some commentators, GPs, especially part-time GPs, are responsible for the downfall of the NHS. Long waits in emergency departments and for ambulances, millions on waiting lists and difficulties seeing a doctor face to face. If only GPs would stop being part time, then all these problems would be solved.

The implication that an entire group of professionals are work-shy by being part timers is akin to the toxic reports of GPs doing nothing during the pandemic. And it is hard to stomach these comments when the reality for primary care is one of daily firefighting: limitless amounts of work without the resources to match.

As a part-time GP, I work 3, sometimes 4 days a week. That's six regular sessions in 3 days. I qualified as a GP over 10 years ago and the job has changed enormously in that time, in terms of intensity, pressures and expectations. There are only so many hours in the day, and many GP consultations now routinely spill over the allocated 10 minutes, as GPs deal with multiple complex issues.

In terms of workload, in particular the administrative burden, eight clinical sessions from 20 years ago together is probably the equivalent of about five sessions now.[191]

But what does a 'session' or 'full time' actually mean?

The annual GP Worklife Survey showed in 2022 that the average GP is working 6.3 half day sessions each week, totalling an average of 38.4 hours.[192] Despite NHS digital stating that 'full-time equivalent (FTE) is calculated based upon a 37.5 hour working week',[193] a six-session GP is typically branded a part timer. The BMA model GP contract defines full time as 37.5 hours a week, breaking it down into nine notional sessions of 4 hours 10 minutes.[194]

To put this into perspective, an average 9–5 full-time work week, Monday to Friday, with an hour for lunch, works out at 35 hours a week. Many of the 'part-time' GPs surveyed were clocking up 37.5 hours with ease.[195] To unpick this a little more, a half day 'session' in general practice has traditionally been defined as 4 hours 10 minutes. Most GPs will now tell you that the workload has become so intense that this has now stretched to 6 or 7 hours, meaning a session has essentially become a full day's work.

The Sunday Times reported these figures with the opening line: 'Nearly a fifth of GPs work an average of only 26 hours per week as half of all patients struggle to get through to their family doctor.'[196]

As a Pulse editorial pointed out, this headline is based on the 20 per cent of the profession doing the fewest number of hours. And it's still a mere 9 hours less than a normal full-time job.[197] Many of this '20 per cent' often have other roles outside the surgery, not accounted for in the figures – roles which in many cases are actually mandated by the government such as commissioning roles, leading PCNs or LMC work.

As part of DAUK's GP crisis campaign, we gathered stories from frontline general practice and heard of 14-hour days and 60 plus patient contacts a day, which is way above the 25 patient contacts per day considered safe.

If GPs are working 12–14-hour days, then they need to proclaim it to allow clear and transparent discussion. This is three sessions within one working day. We need to define our hours and not accept endless unpaid overtime, or else we will continue to burn out GPs, whose work will remain unrecognised.

I'm now the archetypal female part-time GP. I have two young children and work part time so I can be a mum. Quite frankly, in the current climate, I would be working part time if I didn't have children, and there shouldn't be an obligation for GPs to have to justify reasons for their work patterns. The NHS is not the army, and its staff are not conscripted. At any point, we can make the decision to take the skills we have worked hard to attain and seek employment outside the NHS, where working life is less stressful and more lucrative.

Three of my sessions each week are dedicated purely to admin; I action results and letters coming into the practice. The simple fact that this is needed – hours of a GP's time spent not actually consulting with patients but doing paperwork – shows how much of a strain the unseen admin places on an already stretched system. Initiatives such as advice and guidance (A&G) and e-consults have increased GP workload by adding an extra layer of patient contact. (A&G involves GPs messaging specialist teams for advice and before this was available, the specialist teams would see and deal with patients themselves.) The workload shift from secondary care to general practice is immense, and changes to enable hospital teams to generate their own prescriptions, investigations, medical certificates and interdepartmental referrals would ease so much of this unresourced extra workload passed to GP teams, many who feel they are being used as 'community house officers'.

The 'lazy part-time GP' narrative needs to be quashed. Not only are we being denigrated for being part timers, but 38 hours a week is not part time. In fact, any family doctor who is working more than this is working more than full time and is at risk of burnout. We need to speak up for our profession so that the public are aware. Part-time, flexible working for GPs, and the wider NHS, needs to be embraced rather than derided, to improve both recruitment and retention of staff, which is ultimately better for patient care.

Over to you – Solutions to the GP crisis in a nutshell

This is where you can help. It would be fantastic if this book could be used to create some positive change. Compiled below are some suggested solutions to some of the problems that both general practice and the wider NHS are facing, which have been discussed at length throughout the book. These are summarised in actionable bullet points below.

Once you have finished reading this book, instead of letting it gather dust, we urge you to pass it on to your local member of parliament (member of the Senedd Cymru/member of the Scottish Parliament) and ask them to read the stories shared by frontline staff, patients and family members. Ask them to visit their local GP practices and find out just what is going on locally and what NHS staff in their constituencies need to do to make the service better for patients. Encourage your local library or school to stock this book.

It is time to invest in the service, to push aside party politics and for our leaders to establish an all-party parliamentary group to work towards fixing the NHS. General practice is the bedrock of the NHS, and, sadly, if general practice fails, then so does the wider NHS.

Many of the initiatives suggested below can be taken up locally, while many are solutions which need to be pushed through by the government. It's divided into digestible sections, being aware there is much overlap in who can action change.

For the government
Remove the NHS from the political agenda. Form a cross-party group to focus on the NHS and health care, comprised of MPs from all parties, alongside experienced healthcare professionals, so that each time an election rolls around, the service is not at the mercy of politicians promising polished soundbites. Each new government generally brings about a costly, unevidenced reorganisation of the service. Step back from this and focus on the problems rather than winning votes.

Address workforce retention. The leaky bucket analogy holds true here. There's no point continuing to fill a leaking NHS with more trainee doctors if they are haemorrhaging out of the system once qualified. Continue reading for more ideas on how to do this.

Address red tape. Much of the box ticking in general practice adds little to patient care and detracts from our core work. Additional pressures on staff can be reduced by re-examining the need for CQC inspections, appraisals and revalidation.

Streamline NHS technology. Secondary care should have the same digital technology enabled as primary care, to avoid workload being passed to GPs This would include using interactive short messaging service (SMS or 'text messaging') – to allow hospital teams to send sick notes and results to patients – and introducing an electronic prescribing service (EPS). Within primary care, so much time would be saved if IT systems didn't regularly crash or take time to load.

Put the NHS on the school curriculum. Patients can't be blamed for their navigation of a system that many health professionals struggle with.

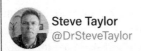

Steve Taylor
@DrSteveTaylor

Looking for a tradesperson

Can anyone recommend someone for me?
Can you do this job?

I am looking for a contract with a plumber/electrician/painter/
plasterer/odd job person (you need to have ALL these skills) to
provide an annual contract service for me.

I am willing to pay £150 per year for this contract – no more. No
call-out fee and I can call you as many times as I like, for repairs,
even if I have ignored your advice previously.

You will need to be available between 0800-1830hrs on weekdays.
Outside of these times, I am willing to pay an additional £18 per year
to have access to an emergency service to sort me out until my
contracted tradesperson is available.

Again, no call-out fees.

I will only take those tradespeople who have done 10 years of
training and prove via rigorous annual assessment by peers that
they remain up-to-date, and ethical, and won't cheat me.

Sounds incredible, doesn't it?

How many of you will find a tradesperson like that willing to sign up?

Most would laugh down the phone at you.

WELL, THAT IS EXACTLY WHAT YOUR GP PRACTICE GETS
TO PROVIDE YOU SERVICE FOR A YEAR, AND WHAT
IS EXPECTED OF THEM.

Think about that, the next time you are annoyed you can't get an
appointment and wonder why so many GPs and their teams are
leaving the NHS.

My generation have grown up with the message to 'get checked out' and see your GP for every ill. Education about minor/self-limiting illness and health promotion should be part of the school curriculum, along with teaching on what the NHS is, how it works, and how to access care, for example when its more appropriate to go to A&E or a GP. Follow the DAUK for more ideas on how to implement this (see below).

Value the workforce so they want to stay. NHS staff are its greatest resource. At a government level this would involve:
- Committing to full pay restoration for the wider NHS workforce.
- End hospital parking charges. The pandemic proved it could be done.
- Address the blame culture.
- Provide the next generation of doctors with access to full maintenance loans to avoid them graduating with six-figure sums of debt.
- Streamline the visa system for international medical staff who are often prevented from taking up NHS jobs due to Home Office bureaucracy.
- Scrap the immigration surcharge. One in four doctors working in the NHS come to provide a service from outside of the UK and without them the service would collapse. Doctors in the UK on a visa essentially pay for NHS services twice – through taxation and through this surcharge.

For NHS/GP leaders and staff

Rebrand the profession. Since 2019, the GMC has supported calls from both the RCGP and the BMA to recognise GPs as specialists.[198] Renaming GPs as 'consultants in family medicine', or similar, has been debated for some time, and the profession struggle to agree. Name changes are confusing, and with so many health professionals calling themselves consultants these days, it isn't always clear to patients who they are seeing, and this is important. Whether or not we rename GPs as consultants, we should be clear about the job GPs do. GPs *are* specialists in being generalists. There needs to be recognition GPs are leading large teams, dealing with more complexity, and supervising colleagues.

Redefine GP working hours. If your two 4-hour sessions have both lasted 6 hours, then you've done three sessions not two. Speak up for the unseen work, staff have survived on goodwill for too long.

Cap GP's workload. BMA safe working in general practice supports GPs to limit contacts to 25 per day to prioritise safe patient care. Medicine has changed and GP consultations are more complex now than they were 75 years ago. Our systems need to adapt to this reality.

Embrace flexible working. A remote or part-time GP who isn't burnt out is better than no GP at all.

Deal with un-resourced workload. With pressures as they are, GP teams have no capacity to do non-contractual work passed from elsewhere (e.g. secondary care requests). Use your LMC for local practices to work together with a united stance on responding to non-contractual work, use BMA template letters (see below). Meet with secondary care leaders to address the default 'ask your GP' stance – for example hospitals asking patients to contact their GP to expedite a hospital appointment takes up hours of GP time each week – and makes little difference. Hospital doctors have annual inductions and GPs need to be part of these so new staff are aware of the interaction between primary and secondary care and the local pressures. Systems need to change so GPs can focus on core work instead of drowning in external work.

BMA template letters to challenge these requests are available here: <*www.bma.org.uk/advice-and-support/gp-practices/managing-workload/ pushing-back-on-inappropriate-workload*>.

Simplify referral processes. A GP referral should be a straightforward message to the relevant provider that according to the GP's professional judgement, their patient's needs can no longer be entirely met within the community. Ten-page referral forms and rejected referrals for arbitrary reasons add to delays for patient care and detract from our core work. Liaise with secondary care to re-examine the need for these proformas, instead of a concise letter containing relevant information, or better still, see below.

Streamline NHS technology. Secondary care should have the same digital technology enabled as primary care to avoid workload being passed to GPs and allow instant information sharing. This would work both ways: it would avoid lengthy referral proformas if specialists can see full medical histories and GP teams waiting weeks to get hospital discharge letters.

Value the workforce so they want to stay. This often works better in general practice than it does in the larger institutions of secondary care, and will look different in every workplace, but ensuring that the basics of Maslow's hierarchy of needs are met is even more important when the pressure is on. Most healthcare professionals will happily manage a degree of workload pressure if in return they feel appreciated.

Address the blame culture. 'Learn not blame' is one of the central campaigns of DAUK, launched in Parliament in 2018 to create a culture change within the NHS to improve both patient safety and the wellbeing of healthcare staff.[199] The campaign calls for a system that learns from errors rather than undue blame being diverted upon individuals and that everyone working in the NHS should be empowered to do what they can within their own sphere of influence to ensure safer patient care. For example, raising concerns about staff shortages with managers. The recent shocking case of serial killing neonatal nurse Lucy Letby sadly shows how much work still needs to be done. In August

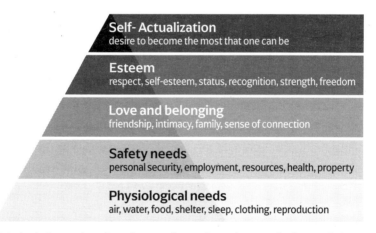

Maslow's hierarchy of needs is a theory formed in 1943 by psychologist Abraham Maslow. He outlined that humans have needs that must be met ranging from the most basic physiological needs (food, water, sleep…) to the most complex needs. Maslow outlined how people will first be consumed by their basic needs before being able to meet more advanced needs. For example, a doctor working a 12-hour shift, without access to food or a toilet break is unlikely to be motivated to do an excellent job.

2023,[200] Letby was sentenced to life in prison for the murder of seven babies and the attempted murder of six others who were under her care. Consultant paediatricians who raised concerns about Letby were silenced, accused of bullying and threatened with GMC referral by managers at the Countess of Chester Hospital. The CQC inspected the hospital during Letby's time, rating it as 'good'. The regulation of health service managers has been recommended to ensure standards are set in the same way they are for clinicians.[201]

You and your GP

Here are some tips on how to make the most of your GP appointments from the perspective of the GP.

Do you need a GP appointment?

Many GPs' appointments are taken up by people with a few hours of a sore throat or similar problems which will settle by themselves with time and self-care. The human body is designed to cure a lot of things itself, especially minor infections. Similarly, a lot of chronic health problems could be improved by a holistic look at lifestyle. For example, one of my patients once casually told me about the two bottles of vodka she was getting through each weekend without considering that it was a problem. Children are routinely offered sweets and processed food with little thought about the health consequences. Putting the NHS and health literacy on the school curriculum would go a long way to addressing some of these presentations, hopefully giving people the confidence to be able to manage minor illness with self-care and to engage in healthier ways of living. Campaigns to warn of the dangers of missing cancers or sepsis have done a lot to raise awareness, and save lives, but they have also increased anxiety and led to people seeking care earlier when often self-care is sufficient.

For more information on dealing with minor illness see: <*https:// thepracticeofhealth.nhs.wales/clinics-services/self-help-care/minor-common-ailments/*>.

Let the practice team signpost you

Many problems can be managed effectively by the wider practice team, or the wider NHS, and it may be appropriate to be 'signposted' elsewhere. If you're chasing up a hospital referral, call the secretary at the hospital first. If you need a blood pressure check, many surgeries have pods to do this at reception or it can be done in a pharmacy. If you need a referral, often you can self-refer for services such as physiotherapy, counselling or for antenatal midwife-led care. If your problem is with your teeth or gums, then please see a dentist. Minor injuries can be dealt with by minor injury units, and remember, general practice is not an emergency service. Conditions such as heart attacks, strokes and severe bleeding need A&E. Other ways to access medical advice:

- Online via *<www.nhs.uk>* or by calling NHS 111.
- Visiting a pharmacy.
- Optometrists (opticians) are much more skilled at dealing with eye problems than most GPs, and in England, a relatively new service enables patients to seek help with eye problems directly from their local optician instead of their GP. See: *<https://primaryeyecare. co.uk>* for more information.

Set the agenda

GP appointments last 10 minutes, sometimes 15, depending on the practice. If you have two problems to discuss, either book a double appointment in advance, or mention your agenda from the outset so problems can be prioritised, rather than saying on the way out 'while I'm here, there are just a couple of other things'. Bringing long lists of problems has become common, but it's not possible to deal with a list in 10 minutes. It may be that several appointments are needed to give each problem due attention. Try to raise the serious problems first (i.e. chest pain is more urgent than a fungal toenail).

Get to the point

Precise timescales are more helpful than vague ones, and concise descriptions of your symptoms are helpful. Telling your GP 'I've got a chest infection' is not as useful as telling them the symptoms that are bothering you (i.e. 'cough, breathlessness, wheeze,' and so on). Be honest. Your GP will understand that some problems are embarrassing but if they don't have the full story, it makes helping you more difficult. Tell your GP what you're worried about so they can address your concerns directly. GPs look for certain 'red flag' symptoms that make them concerned about diagnoses such as cancers, and if your history doesn't raise these red flags, they may not even bring up the C word.

However, if this is your overwhelming reason for the visit and you don't mention it, you may leave the room just as worried as when you came in. Tell your GP.

Realistic expectations

It is unlikely that your GP can solve everything in one visit. Many people have several ongoing problems, or complex needs, and ongoing monitoring, investigations and further appointments with the wider practice team may be needed. If you are referred to secondary care, then you may need to wait some time for this. You should always feel listened to however, and please ask questions, ask about timescales and if the outcome is different to what you expected from the consultation, talking about why may be helpful.

Medical records

Many patients take it for granted that their entire medical history is 'all there in the computer'. Sadly, this may not always be the case, especially if you are new to a practice. It can take some time for notes to be transferred. Keeping a record yourself of your medical problems and medications can be extremely useful in situations like this, as well as if you are travelling overseas. Many new healthcare apps are available to do this. Many more patients are accessing tests privately which are not sent to NHS GPs, so collating all your medical information in one place is useful.

Symptom diaries

Keeping a diary of symptoms and patterns can be helpful for some problems. For example, if the problem is irregular periods, using a period tracker app can be invaluable in tracking symptoms and seeing patterns. For migraines, keeping track of triggers can be useful and can jog your memory. Keeping track of what you have tried yourself and what helped is also useful (e.g. 'I took ibuprofen and it helped').

Think about clothing

If you are coming to have a physical examination, then think about wearing clothes that are quick and easy to remove. If it takes 3 minutes to undress and redress, that's a third of your appointment wasted.

'Get a note from your GP'

GPs have become the go-to stop for every problem, and one request that takes up a lot of GP time is for letters. Many of these requests range from the unnecessary to the absurd, with many requests attempting to shift responsibility for potential adverse consequences away from themselves (for example, requests to certify fitness to [insert activity]). GPs already do more work than they are paid to do, and any time spent doing non-funded extras like this, is time taken away from core work. If you have been asked by an organisation to 'get a note from your GP', then, firstly, question the need for it. Common requests include notes for school absence, exam exemptions or medication use at school (parents/guardians are responsible and can provide a note themselves). Fitness to drive or fly requests are common and should be done by doctors with appropriate expertise. The DVLA have dedicated doctors to do this. Similarly, occupational health assessments are the responsibility of employers and not something that should default to the GP. Letters like this are private work so if your own GP does agree to proceed, then expect to be charged.

The following website provides an excellent resource on this topic, with links to information on fit notes and how to self-certify: <*www. ganfyd.org*>.

Courtesy requests

- Please be on time. GPs are trying to offer the same courtesy and run to time, but if they are not, this is usually because they are either dealing with a medical emergency, discussing a serious diagnosis or trying to manage the expectations of patients bringing multiple problems to the consultations. Thank you for your patience.
- Please don't answer your mobile phone during your appointment.
- Be aware practices have a zero-tolerance approach to abuse.
- If you realise you can't make your appointment, cancel it. Hundreds of appointments are wasted each year because of DNAs ('did not attend').
- Remember to order repeat medications in time to avoid the request becoming an urgent one when the medication runs out.
- Please don't ask your GP to deal with the problems of a relative during your appointment. Please book a separate appointment for them.

Media messaging

This isn't appointment related, but patients will try to see their GP to ask about the latest health story or scare, and throughout this book we've described how deflating it has been for GPs to shoulder the negative press. GPs need a better PR team. Questioning the messages given by mainstream media should be encouraged, with the knowledge that most media outlets have a political stance that influences their reporting. In the summer of 2023, a tabloid newspaper announced that 'one in six people have waited at least 2 weeks to see a GP in England in the past year.'[202]

'Oh dear,' responded commentator Roy Lilley. 'More shame on the NHS. Another kicking for GPs. Apart from the obvious that five in six people are getting to see their GP very promptly.'

It transpires that the article was regurgitated from a press release from the Liberal Democrats. Most headlines are written as a form of entertainment, written in a simplified or sensational way to get clicks, to a deadline, and the nature of the problems within the NHS cannot be realistically reduced to the limited word count of a front-page article.

Doctors' Association UK (DAUK)

The royalties for this book are going to DAUK, so you may be interested in learning a little more about this important organisation and the vital work they do.

DAUK is a strictly non-profit, volunteer-led campaigning and lobbying organisation made up of UK doctors and medical students. It was founded in 2018 by grassroot doctors in the wake of the case of Hadiza Bawa-Garba, to advocate for the medical profession and a better NHS.[203]

DAUK's GP Committee was formed in 2020, during the pandemic, to speak out about the growing crisis in general practice and respond to frequent negative misinformation from some sections of the media.

Response to our IPSO letter

#GPCrisis

"

Absolutely shocking piece of journalism... the profession is on its knees

Come and sit with me for a day and see my work

Why does the British press hate GPs so much? What's their actual agenda?

I regularly work 5 hours of extra unpaid work everyday

Most difficult year of my career

Thank you DAUK

"

Committee members have volunteered their time for important advocacy work, writing articles, appearing on major news channels, meeting with NHS leaders and briefing MPs, often with other campaign groups such as 'GP Survival'.

DAUK challenged damaging press coverage misrepresenting GPs – their complaint against one such *Telegraph* article to the Independent Press Standards Organisation (IPSO) gathered nearly 3,000 signatures. DAUK also advocates for medical education reform and lobbied for a liveable NHS bursary for students. The team have criticised the GMC's treatment of international and BAME doctors. They were also one of the first health organisations to support the Climate and Ecology Bill and support incentives for a greener NHS. All this in their free time alongside busy NHS jobs.[204]

DAUK set up the **#GPCrisis** tag on social media as a powerful way to share stories and champion GP teams. This book is an extension of this work, aiming to reach non-doctors with a mix of facts, history and personal stories.

You can get involved with DAUK's work and support them over on their website *<www.dauk.org>* and on social media.

List of contributors

Dr Aman Amir
GP partner in Liverpool, author of many novels, university lecturer and magistrate in Manchester.

Dr Neil Barnard
Consultant in emergency and intensive care medicine, now based in South Africa.

Dr Zainab Batool
London-based GP, interim chief medical officer, healthcare consultant, founder and medical device inventor.

Dr Elizabeth Croton
GP based in Birmingham and sessional doctor with NHS Practitioner Health. Dr Croton has held various roles as a GP, writer and member of DAUK's GP Committee.

Dr Paul Evans
GP and chair of Gateshead and South Tyneside Local Medical Committee.

Dr Christine Hunter
Retired NHS GP.

Dr Louise Hyde
GP in Wales.

Dr Neena Jha
GP in Hertfordshire.

Dr Robin Kåss
Doctor in Avonova, the largest private provider of occupational health services in Norway. Dr Kåss trained at Liverpool University before

returning home to work as a GP in Norway. He was deputy minister in the Norwegian Ministry of Health and Care Services (2010), and mayor of the city of Porsgrunn (2015–23). Director of Acute, Emergency and Prehospital care at Telemark Hospital in Telemark, Norway.

Dr Amir Khan

NHS GP in Bradford, senior lecturer and GP trainer. After appearing on Channel 5's *GPs Behind Closed Doors* he went on to become a bestselling author and the resident doctor for ITV's *Lorraine* and *Good Morning Britain*.

Roy Lilley

Health policy analyst, writer, broadcaster and commentator on health care.

Dr Catriona McNicol

GP partner in Yorkshire.

Chris Milligan

Father and widower of Dr Gail Milligan.

Dr Lois Mugleston

GP in Nottingham, GP appraiser, and participates in teaching and training of GPs. Passionate about the prevention of disease, Dr Mugleston was a GP in New Zealand from 2007–15 and owned and ran a practice in semi-rural west Auckland.

Dr Ayan Panja

NHS GP partner in St Albans, Hertfordshire. Dr Panja is a lifestyle medicine educator, author, podcaster, former BBC World News presenter and editorial advisor to NHS Digital.

Ellie Philpotts

Award-winning health journalist, teenage cancer survivor and creative writer.

Dr Eric Rose

Retired NHS GP. Member of the GP Committee of the BMA (1989–2008). Dr Rose played a leading role in the campaign to reform GP out of hours.

Dr Sarah Rushworth
GP in Nova Scotia and assistant professor at Dalhousie University, Halifax, Canada.

Ron Templeton
Retired tutor and lecturer at Liverpool University Medical School. Honorary life president of the Liverpool Medical Students Society.

Dr Lizzie Toberty
GP in Newcastle, GP lead with DAUK.

Dr Ellen Welch
GP in Cumbria, co-chair of DAUK (2022–3).

Dr David Wrigley
GP partner in Carnforth, Lancashire, and deputy chair of the BMA's GP Committee in England.

Glossary

Accident and emergency (A&E)

More correctly known as the emergency department, previously 'casualty', this is the part of a hospital where people go for treatment of urgent medical conditions, such as major injuries from trauma, road traffic accidents or falls from a considerable height; episodes of severe chest pain or severe breathing difficulties; symptoms of a stroke; severe bleeding or burns; or episodes of poisoning. Some A&E departments have a Minor Injury Unit attached to them (in some areas these are on separate locations) which deal with minor injuries such as sprains, minor fractures and head injuries and wounds. For patients, navigating where to go for care is tricky. Some health professionals even find it difficult. The NHS website provides the following advice: *<www.nhs. uk/nhs-services/urgent-and-emergency-care-services/when-to-go-to-ae/>*.

Accident Compensation Corporation (ACC)

New Zealand's accident insurance scheme, which provides cover for accidental injury to all New Zealand residents and temporary visitors to the country.

Additional Roles Reimbursement Scheme (ARRS)

A funding scheme available to PCNs to support recruitment of 'additional roles' including clinical pharmacists, pharmacy technicians, social prescribing link workers, health and wellbeing coaches, care co-ordinators, PAs, first contact physiotherapists, dieticians, podiatrists, occupational therapists, nurse training associates, community paramedics, advanced practitioners, general practice assistants and mental health practitioners.

Advanced nurse practitioner (ACP)

ACPs are experienced registered nurses educated to master's level in advanced practice, who can manage the complete clinical care for their patient within the limits of their clinical competence.

Advice and guidance (A&G)

A communication between GPs/referrers and consultant-led secondary care services carried out electronically, whereby GPs can seek advice or clarification on the care of an NHS patient. NHS England's explanation: *<www.england.nhs.uk/elective-care-transformation/best-practice-solutions/ advice-and-guidance/#:~:text=What%20is%20Advice%20and%20 Guidance,IT%20platforms%20or%20email%20addresses>*.

Agenda for Change clinicians

Agenda for Change is the NHS pay and grading system for most NHS staff. Doctors, dentists, apprentices and some senior managers are excluded from this scheme. Further info: *<https://nursingnotes.co.uk/ agenda-for-change-nhs-pay-bands>*.

British Medical Association (BMA)

Registered trade union for doctors in the UK, which was founded in 1832.

Care Quality Commission (CQC)

An executive non-departmental public body of the Department of Health and Social Care established in 2009 to regulate and inspect health and social care providers in England.

Certificate of Eligibility for GP Registration (CEGPR)

An alternative route to become registered as a GP in the UK. For example, it is the route used by GPs who have qualified overseas to show their training is equivalent.

Clinical commissioning groups (CCGs)

Clinically led statutory NHS bodies responsible for planning and commissioning health care. They replaced PCTs on 1 April 2013 and were dissolved in July 2022, replaced by ICSs.

Clinical nurse specialists (CNS)

Advanced practice registered nurses who have completed a master's or doctoral degree.

Continuing professional development (CPD)
The learning activity doctors need to do to maintain professional standards. Doctors must complete revalidations with the GMC every 5 years. Part of this is providing evidence that CPD has been completed.

Doctors' Association UK (DAUK)
See section above 'Doctors' Association UK (DAUK)'.

Electronic prescribing service (EPS)
The system by which prescribers can electronically send prescriptions to dispensers. The benefit of this is that patients can collect prescriptions directly from a pharmacy without picking up a prescription from their GP first. This also reduces paper use.

General Medical Council (GMC)
The regulator of doctors in the UK. The GMC sets standards, holds a register of doctors and investigates complaints.

General Medical Services (GMS)
The range of health care provided by GPs in the UK. GPs are independent contractors and the NHS holds a contract to provide funding for this work through arrangements known as the General Medical Services contracts. You can read the GP contract page at NHS England here: *<www.england.nhs.uk/gp/investment/gp-contract/>*.

General practices
Small- to medium-sized business whose services are contracted by NHS commissioners to provide generalist medical services in a geographical area.

GP contracts
Further reading on GP contracts/funding: *<www.kingsfund.org.uk/publications/gp-funding-and-contracts-explained>*.

GP partner
GPs who own a stake in the practice business they work in. Some practices are run by individual 'single handed' GPs but most are run as a partnership of two or more, who pool resources such as buildings

and staff. Partners are responsible for meeting the requirements of their contract and sharing the income it provides.

Healthcare Inspectorate Wales (HIW)
The independent regulator of health care in Wales (equivalent to the CQC).

Immigration Health Surcharge (IHS)
Introduced in 2015, the IHS allows migrants to use the NHS. Current fees are £1,035 per person, per year, meaning an adult applying for a 5-year visa to the UK will need to budget £5,175 for this alone.

Integrated care systems (ICS)
ICSs (prior to 2022 these were CCGs) are partnerships of organisations (NHS organisations, local authorities and others) which join together to plan and deliver joined-up health and care services, with the aim to improve health and reduce inequalities across geographical areas.

Local Medical Committee (LMC)
LMCs are local committees representing GPs working within the NHS. They have a statutory duty to represent GPs which was enshrined in law in 1911 and continues as part of the Health and Social Care Act 2012. Each area of the country has an LMC, and GPs are nominated in each locality to represent their peers.

Locum GP
A fully qualified GP who provides temporary assistance to a service. This can be on an ad hoc basis, or long term with more regular hours at the same practice.

NHS Confederation
A membership body for organisations that commission and provide NHS services. Formerly known as the National Association of Health Authorities and Trusts.

Out of hours (OOH)
The period of time when GP surgeries are closed, between 6.30pm to 8am weekdays, weekends and bank holidays.

Performers lists
The performers lists provide a regulatory framework (in addition to the GMC) to ensure medical, dental and ophthalmic practitioners who contract with NHS England are qualified and competent to provide safe and effective primary care services. GPs may only provide NHS primary care services in England if they are on this list.

Physician associate (PA)
PAs are healthcare professionals who work to the medical model and work across both primary and secondary care. PAs were introduced to the UK in 2003 and there are 1,500 now working in hospitals and 1,700 in primary care. They are currently unregulated and work under the supervision of a designated senior doctor. The Faculty of Physician Associates (FPA) says PAs are intended to work 'alongside' doctors, while the BMA GP Committee have emphasised the fact that a PA is not a substitute for a doctor since they do not undertake the same number of years of training. As the BMA states: 'GPs play a particularly important role in diagnosing serious conditions, a task that can be only done with an appropriate level of medical expertise and experience.'

Primary care groups (PCGs)
Now defunct, these were the predecessors to PCTs, CCGs and the current ICSs. They were formed in 1999 to commission health services. They were replaced by PCTs in 2002.

Primary care network (PCN)
Almost all general practices in England are part of a PCN, which is a small group of practices, usually within the same geographical area, that work together under the PCN direct enhanced service (DES) contract to gain some of the benefits of working at scale and access to additional funding.

Primary care trusts (PCTs)
Replaced PCGs in 2002 until they were replaced by CCGs in 2013. PCTs were responsible for commissioning health services.

Private finance initiative (PFI)
Scheme by which public sector projects are financed by private sector investors.

Problem-based learning (PBL)

A student-centred teaching method which uses complex real-world problems to promote student learning.

Royal College of General Practitioners (RCGP)

Professional body for GPs in the UK. The college represents and supports GPs.

Salaried GP

A GP who works as an employee of a GP practice without owning a share in the overall business (like GP partners). Practices running a General Medical Services (GMS) contract are required to offer a British Medical Association (BMA) model salaried employment contract for these staff.

Single-handed GP

A single-handed GP runs their own practice without any other GP partners.

Help for GPs

The Balint Society *www.balint.co.uk/find-a-group/*
Society that enables health professionals to form groups to gain a better understanding of the emotional content of their relationship with patients.

BMA wellbeing resources
www.bma.org.uk/advice-and-support/your-wellbeing
All doctors and medical students can access the BMA's 24/7 counselling line and a host of helpful support services.

British Doctors and Dentists Group *www.bddg.org*
Recovery group for doctors and dentists with addictions.

The Cameron Fund *www.cameronfund.org.uk*
Medical benevolent charity which supports GPs and their dependants suffering from financial hardship.

Canopi *www.canopi.nhs.wales*
Free and confidential mental health support for NHS and social care staff across Wales.

Disabled Doctors Network *www.disableddoctorsnetwork.com*
Support network for chronically ill and disabled doctors.

DocHealth *www.dochealth.org.uk*
Confidential psychotherapy service for all doctors.

Doctors in Distress *www.doctors-in-distress.org.uk*
UK charity protecting the mental health of healthcare workers and preventing suicide.

Doctors' Support Network *www.dsn.org.uk*
Peer support for doctors and medical students with mental health concerns

Domestic Abuse Support for Doctors *www.dasdorguk.wordpress.com*
Support specifically for doctors impacted by domestic abuse.

Frontline 19 *www.frontline19.com*
Established during the Covid-19 pandemic, this service provides psychological support for people working in the NHS and frontline services.

GLADD (The Association of LGBTQ+ Doctors and Dentists) *www.gladd.co.uk*
Offers support, advice and representation to LGBTQ+ doctors, dentists and students.

Health for Health Professionals Wales (HHP Wales) *www.hcpc-uk.org*
Face-to-face counselling service for doctors in Wales.

HSC staff health and wellbeing

https://www.publichealth.hscni.net/covid-19-coronavirus/guidance-hsc-staff-healthcare-workers-and-care-providers/staff-health-and
Psychological helplines for health and social care staff in Northern Ireland.

Long Covid Doctors for Action *www.facebook.com/groups/lcd4a/?ref=share_group_link*
Private support group for GMC registered doctors affected by long covid.

The Louise Tebboth Foundation *www.louisetebboth.org.uk*
Grant giving charity advocating for the prevention of suicide and recognition of the wellbeing of doctors.

Medical Womens Federation *www.medicalwomensfederation.org.uk*
Working to improve the working lives of women doctors.

Melanin Medics *www.melaninmedics.com*
Promotes diversity in medicine and works to increase the representation of African and Caribbean practitioners in medicine.

National Association of Sessional GPs *www.nasgp.org.uk*
Community for GP locums and salaried GPs.

NHS talking and psychological therapies (IAPT services)
www.nhs.uk/mental-health/talking-therapies-medicine-treatments/talking-therapies-and-counselling/nhs-talking-therapies/
Free talking and psychological therapies on the NHS (non-medic specific).

Practitioner Health Programme *www.practitionerhealth.nhs.uk*
Award winning, free and confidential NHS service for doctors and dentists with issues relating to mental health concerns or addiction problems, in particular where these might affect their work.

Project 5 *https://www.project5.org*
Free psychological support sessions for health and care workers.

Protect *www.protect-advice.org.uk*
Free, confidential advice for whistleblowers.

Royal College of Psychiatrists' Support Service
www.rcpsych.ac.uk/members/workforce-wellbeing-hub/psychiatrists-support-service
Provides peer support by telephone to psychiatrists experiencing work or personal difficulties. They also have a group for doctors affected by suicide.

Royal Medical Benevolent Fund *www.rmbf.org*
Support for doctors and their families through all stages of their career. Help ranges from financial assistance in the form of grants and loans to a telephone befriending scheme.

Royal Medical Foundation *www.royalmedicalfoundation.org*
Benevolent charity which helps UK medical practitioners and their dependants in financial hardship.

Second Victim Support *www.secondvictim.co.uk*
Support for healthcare workers involved in a patient safety incident and its investigation.

Sick Doctors Trust *www.sick-doctors-trust.co.uk*
Support for doctors, dentists and medical students who are concerned about their use of drugs or alcohol.

Society for Assistance of Medical Families *www.samf.org.uk*
Membership society assisting doctors and their families during times of hardship.

Surviving in Scrubs *www.survivinginscrubs.co.uk*
Campaign to end sexism, sexual harassment and sexual assault in healthcare by sharing lived experiences.

Workforce Specialist Service
www.wellbeinghub.scot/the-workforce-specialist-service-wss/
Mental health service for health and social care staff in Scotland.

You Okay Doc? *www.youokaydoc.org.uk*
Mental health and wellbeing charity for doctors.

Further reading

This list is not comprehensive. It acts as a suggested list of books which may be of interest.

Berger, John, *A Fortunate Man: The Story of a Country Doctor* (London: Allen Lane, 1967).

Bulgakov, Mikhail, *A Country Doctor's Notebook*, trans. Michael Glenny (London: Vintage Classics, 2010).

Helman, Cecil, *Suburban Shaman* (London: Hammersmith Press Limited, 2006).

Holmes, Rachel, *Scanty Particulars: The Life of Dr James Barry* (London: Viking, 2002).

Morland, Polly, *A Fortunate Woman: A Country Doctor's Story* (London: Picador, 2022).

Orlans, David et al., *What's in a Story? Lessons from Reflections in General Practice* (Solihull: Hampton-In-Arden Publishing, 2017).

Widgery, David, *Some Lives: A GP's East End* (London: Simon & Schuster Ltd, 1992).

Williams, Ian, *The Bad Doctor: The Troubled Life and Times of Dr Iwan James* (London: Myriad Editions, 2014).

Endnotes

1 E. Welch, 'NHS at 75: I dread telling people I'm a GP – we need a government that values us', GPonline <*www.gponline.com/nhs-75-i-dread-telling-people-im-gp-need-government-values-us/article/1828827*>.

2 'Activity in the NHS', The King's Fund (2020) <*www.kingsfund.org.uk/projects/nhs-in-a-nutshell/NHS-activity*>.

3 G. Rivett, '(1948–57): Establishing the National Health Service', Nuffield Trust <*www.nuffieldtrust.org.uk/chapter/1948-1957-establishing-the-national-health-service*>.

4 'Bevan's speech to the Executive Councils Association 7 October 1948', Socialist Health Association <*www.sochealth.co.uk/national-health-service/the-sma-and-the-foundation-of-the-national-health-service-dr-leslie-hilliard-1980/aneurin-bevan-and-the-foundation-of-the-nhs/bevans-speech-to-the-executive-councils-association-7-october-1948/*>.

5 'Pressures in general practice data analysis', BMA (2023) <*www.bma.org.uk/advice-and-support/nhs-delivery-and-workforce/pressures/pressures-in-general-practice-data-analysis*>.

6 'Causes of death over 100 years', Office of National Statistics, 18 September 2017 <*www.ons.gov.uk/peoplepopulationandcommunity/birthsdeathsandmarriages/deaths/articles/causesofdeathover100years/2017-09-18*>.

7 H. L. Smith, '"Hunger, filth, fear and death" – remembering life before the NHS', *New Statesman*, October 2014 <*www.newstatesman.com/long-reads/2014/10/hunger-filth-fear-and-death-remembering-life-nhs*>.

8 'Health care before the NHS', Nuffield Trust <*www.nuffieldtrust.org.uk/chapter/inheritance#introduction-the-inheritance-of-the-nhs*>.

9 'Report of the inter-departmental committee on remuneration of general practitioners', Spens Committee, Cmd 6810 (London: HMSO, 1946).

10 John Fry, 'General practice and primary health care: 1940s–1980s', Nuffield Trust <*www.nuffieldtrust.org.uk/files/2017-01/general-practice-web-final.pdf*>.

11 'The evolving role and nature of general practice in England', The King's Fund (2011) <*www.kingsfund.org.uk/sites/default/files/field/field_related_document/gp-inquiry-report-evolving-role-nature-2mar11.pdf*>.

12 R. Lilley, 'Gone…' (2022) <*https://myemail.constantcontact.com/Wonder-where-it-s-gone.html?soid=1102665899193&aid=soKoFtHjUpM*>.

13 S. Taylor, *Good General Practice* (London: Oxford University Press, 1954).

14 E. Anthony, 'The GP at the crossroads', *British Medical Journal*, 1 (1950), 1077–9.

15 J. S. Collings, 'General practice in England today: a reconnaissance', *The Lancet*, 255/6604 (1950), 555–85.

16 H. Danckwerts, 'Remuneration of general practitioners', *The Lancet*, 259/6709 (1952), 662.

17 J. Tudor Hart, 'A New Kind of Doctor 4 New Ideas in Old Structures', Socialist Health Association, 14 October 1988 <*www.sochealth.co.uk/1988/10/14/new-kind-doctor-4-new-ideas-old-structures/*>.

18 E. Philpotts, 'GPs should be rebranded as "consultants in family medicine", say LMCs', GPonline <*www.gponline.com/gps-rebranded-consultants-family-medicine-say-lmcs/article/1823297*>.

19 E. Rose, 'The True History of GP Out of Hours Services', A Better NHS, 10 May 2013 <*https://abetternhs.net/2013/05/10/true-history/*>.

20 'Raising Standards for Patients. New partnerships in Out-of-Hours-Care', Department of Health (2000) *www.esydave.com/uploads/1/4/0/9/14097905/____carson_2000_ooh_review.pdf.*

21 House of Commons, 'Health – Fifth Report' (2004) <*https://publications.parliament.uk/pa/cm200304/cmselect/cmhealth/697/69702.htm*>.

22 R. Fisher, 'NHS winter pressures: How well prepared is the NHS in England?', The Health Foundation, 8 December 2017 <*www.health.org.uk/blogs/nhs-winter-pressures-how-well-prepared-is-the-nhs-in-england*>.

23 'NHS 111', Nuffield Trust <*www.nuffieldtrust.org.uk/resource/nhs-111*>.

24 E. Wilkinson, 'GPs call for suspension of NHS 111 referrals into overstretched practices', Pulse, 26 November 2021 <*www.pulsetoday.co.uk/news/urgent-care/gps-call-for-suspension-of-nhs-111-referrals-into-overstretched-practices/*>.

25 'NHS hospital trusts paying hundreds of millions in interest to private firms', *Guardian*, 25 October 2022 <*www.theguardian.com/politics/2022/oct/25/nhs-hospital-trusts-paying-hundreds-of-millions-in-interest-to-private-firms*>.

26 'Some hospitals are spending more on PFI debt than they are on drugs', *New Statesman*, May 2022 <*www.newstatesman.com/spotlight/healthcare/2022/05/pfi-repayments-are-costing-some-hospitals-twice-as-much-as-drugs*>.

27 'GP at Hand is threatening general practice across the UK', Pulse, 20 June 2018 <*www.pulsetoday.co.uk/views/politics/gp-at-hand-is-threatening-general-practice-across-the-uk/*>.

28 I. Kilpatrick, 'Management consultancy in healthcare—time for some independent action?', *British Medical Journal*, 19 July 2021 <*https://blogs.bmj.com/bmj/2021/07/19/management-consultancy-in-healthcare-time-for-some-independent-action/*>.

29 D. Wrigley, 'GPs aren't private companies, but the private takeover is nearing' Open Democracy, 10 September 2014 <*www.opendemocracy.net/en/ournhs/gps-arent-private-companies-but-private-takeover-is-nearing/*>.

30 C. Ham, 'The rise and decline of the NHS in England 2000–20: How political failure led to the crisis in the NHS and social care', The King's Fund, April 2023 <*www.kingsfund.org.uk/sites/default/files/2023-04/Rise_and_Decline_of_the_NHS_April_2023.pdf*>.

31 'A high performing NHS? Review of progress 1997–2010', The King's Fund, April 2010 <*www.kingsfund.org.uk/sites/default/files/summary-high-performing-nhs-*

progress-review-1997-2010-ruth-thorlby-jo-maybin-kings-fund-april-2010_0.pdf>.

32 'Learning from tragedy, keeping patients safe: Overview of the government's action programme in response to the recommendations of the Shipman Inquiry' (2007) <*https://assets.publishing.service.gov.uk/government/uploads/system/uploads/attachment_data/file/228886/7014.pdf>*.

33 'A high-performing NHS? Review of progress 1997–2010', The King's Fund (2010) <*www.kingsfund.org.uk/sites/default/files/summary-high-performing-nhs-progress-review-1997-2010-ruth-thorlby-jo-maybin-kings-fund-april-2010_0.pdf>*.

34 'What is happening to life expectancy in England', The King's Fund (2022) <*www.kingsfund.org.uk/publications/whats-happening-life-expectancy-england>*.

35 P. Whitaker, 'How to save the NHS', *New Statesman*, January 2023 <*www.newstatesman.com/politics/health/2023/01/how-to-save-the-nhs>*

36 P. Whitaker, 'How to save the NHS', *New Statesman*, January 2023 <*www.newstatesman.com/politics/health/2023/01/how-to-save-the-nhs>*.

37 'The challenge facing the NHS in England in 2021', *British Medical Journal*, 31 December 2022, 371: m4973 <*www.bmj.com/content/371/bmj.m4973>*.

38 O. Jones, 'Britain's excess death rate is at a disastrous high – and the causes go far beyond Covid-19', *Guardian*, 15 January 2023 <*www.theguardian.com/commentisfree/2023/jan/15/britain-excess-death-rate-covid-nhs-cost-of-living>*.

39 J. Berger, *A Fortunate Man: The Story of a Country Doctor* (London: Allen Lane, 1967).

40 G. Feder, 'A Fortunate Man: still the most important book about general practice ever written', *British Journal of General Practice* (2005), 246–7 <*https://bjgp.org/content/bjgp/55/512/246.full.pdf>*.

41 P. Morland, *A Fortunate Woman: A Country Doctor's Story* (London: Picador, 2022).

42 Tim Benson, 'Why general practitioners use computers and hospital doctors do not', *British Medical Journal* (2002), 325: 1086 <*www.bmj.com/content/325/7372/1086>*.

43 B. Ireland, 'Unsafe and unsustainable', BMA, 11 July 2023 <*www.bma.org.uk/news-and-opinion/unsafe-and-unsustainable>*.

44 Many of Philip Tetlock's publications can be accessed online <*www.sas.upenn.edu/tetlock/publications>*.

45 'NHS England's 19 March update to GP practices on Covid-19', Pulse, 19 March 2020 <*www.pulsetoday.co.uk/resource/coronavirus/nhs-englands-19-march-update-to-gp-practices-on-covid-19/>*.

46 K. Cooper, 'Most doctors still lack protective equipment, finds survey', BMA, 7 April 2020 <*www.bma.org.uk/news-and-opinion/most-doctors-still-lack-protective-equipment-finds-survey>*.

47 'Remembering the UK doctors who have died of covid-19', *British Medical Journal* <*www.bmj.com/covid-memorial>*.

48 S. Hodes and A. Majjeed, 'Building a sustainable infrastructure for covid-19 vaccinations long term', *British Medical Journal* (2021), 373 <*www.bmj.com/*

content/373/bmj.n1578>.

49 'Appointments in General Practice', NHS Digital, 29 April 2021 <*https:// digital.nhs.uk/data-and-information/publications/statistical/appointments-in-general-practice/march-2021*>.

50 'Appointments in General Practice', NHS Digital, 29 October 2020 <*https://digital.nhs.uk/data-and-information/publications/statistical/appointments-in-general-practice/september-2020*>.

51 'GP access during COVID-19: a review of our evidence: April 2019–December 2020', healthwatch, 22 March 2021 <*www.healthwatch.co.uk/report/2021-03-22/gp-access-during-covid-19*>.

52 A. Pearson, 'GPs are improving their work-life balance while worsening the life-death balance of everyone else', *Telegraph*, 24 August 2021 <*www.telegraph.co.uk/columnists/2021/08/24/gps-improving-work-life-balance-worsening-life-death-balance/*>.

53 'The media's anti-GP agenda', Pulse, 2 February 2021 <*www.pulsetoday.co.uk/analysis/cover-feature/the-medias-anti-gp-agenda/*>.

54 'NHS England sends GPs "reminder" they must offer face-to-face appointments', Pulse, 13 September 2020 <*www.pulsetoday.co.uk/news/coronavirus/nhs-england-sends-gps-reminder-they-must-offer-face-to-face-appointments/*>.

55 C. Potter, 'Practice attacked with anti-GP graffiti', Pulse, 26 October 2021 <*www.pulsetoday.co.uk/news/practice-life/practice-attacked-with-anti-gp-graffiti/*>.

56 N. Bostock, 'How a GP practice kept services running after a suspected arson attack', GPonline, 5 February 2021 <*www.gponline.com/gp-practice-kept-services-running-suspected-arson-attack/article/1706583*>.

57 L. Haynes, 'NHS England's top GP apologises after "offensive" face-to-face appointments letter', GPonline, 15 September 2020 <*www.gponline.com/nhs-englands-top-gp-apologises-offensive-face-to-face-appointments-letter/article/1694434*>.

58 A. Blakey, 'Urgent notice as GP surgery remains closed after "attack on staff"', *Manchester Evening News*, 20 September 2021 <*www.manchestereveningnews.co.uk/news/greater-manchester-news/urgent-notice-gp-surgery-remains-21616143*>.

59 M. Smith, 'GP receptionists punched and racially abused by patients who can't get appointments', Wales Online, 28 September 2021 <*www.walesonline.co.uk/news/health/gps-surgery-doctors-appointments-crisis-21696123*>.

60 E. Bower, 'My GP wife worked herself to death – something needs to change', GPonline, 19 October 2022 <*www.gponline.com/gp-wife-worked-herself-death—something-needs-change/article/1802504*>.

61 'Mental illness and suicide Nov 22 Practitioner Health and Doctors in Distress', NHS Practitioner Health (2022) <*www.practitionerhealth.nhs.uk/mental-illness-and-suicide*>..

62 'Mental illness and suicide Nov 22 Practitioner Health and Doctors in Distress', NHS Practitioner Health (2022) <*www.practitionerhealth.nhs.uk/mental-illness-and-suicide*>.

63 E. Croton, 'GPs are not lazy – we are working harder than ever', metro. co.uk, 10 September 2021 <*https://metro.co.uk/2021/09/10/gps-are-not-lazy-we-are-*

working-harder-than-ever-15233990/>.

64 A. Pearson, 'GPs are improving their work-life balance while worsening the life-death balance of everyone else', *Telegraph*, 24 August 2021 *<www.telegraph.co.uk/columnists/2021/08/24/gps-improving-work-life-balance-worsening-life-death-balance/>.*

65 S. Taylor, X (formerly Twitter) account *<https://twitter.com/DrSteveTaylor>.*

66 'Pressures in general practice data analysis', BMA (2023) *<www.bma.org.uk/advice-and-support/nhs-delivery-and-workforce/pressures/pressures-in-general-practice-data>.*

67 S. Hoddinott and N. Davies, 'Performance Tracker 2022: General practice', Institute for Government, 17 October 2022 *<www.instituteforgovernment.org.uk/performance-tracker-2022/general-practice>.*

68 'Pressures in general practice data analysis', BMA (2023).

69 'Pressures in general practice data analysis', BMA (2023).

70 'NHS Payments to General Practice, England 2021/22', NHS Digital, 24 November 2022 *<https://digital.nhs.uk/data-and-information/publications/statistical/nhs-payments-to-general-practice/england-2021-22>.*

71 'Pressures in general practice data analysis', BMA (2023).

72 A. Gregory, 'NHS test and trace failed its main objective says spending watchdog', *Guardian*, 27 October 2021 *<https://amp.theguardian.com/world/2021/oct/27/nhs-test-and-trace-failed-its-main-objective-says-spending-watchdog>.*

73 'NHS backlog data analysis', BMA (2023) *<www.bma.org.uk/advice-and-support/nhs-delivery-and-workforce/pressures/nhs-backlog-data-analysis>.*

74 'Children waiting two years for mental health support', BBC, 9 March 2023 *<www.bbc.co.uk/news/articles/cw40458j0xdo>.*

75 'NHS backlog data analysis', BMA (2023).

76 C. Baker, 'NHS Key Statistics: England', 19 July 2023 *<https://researchbriefings.files.parliament.uk/documents/CBP-7281/CBP-7281.pdf>.*

77 B. Odebiyi et al., 'Eleventh National GP Worklife Survey 2021', PRUComm, 13 April 2021 *<https://prucomm.ac.uk/eleventh-national-gp-worklife-survey-2021.html>.*

78 'Eleventh National GP Worklife Survey 2021', PRUComm, 19 April 2022 *<https://prucomm.ac.uk/eleventh-national-gp-worklife-survey-2021.html>.*

79 'Eleventh National GP Worklife Survey 2021', PRUComm, 19 April 2022.

80 'The GP Patient Survey' (2023) *<https://gp-patient.co.uk>.*

81 'Fear of legal action impacting on way GPs practise', MPS, 21 December 2017 *<www.medicalprotection.org/uk/articles/fear-of-legal-action-impacting-on-way-gps-practise>.*

82 Toombes vs Mitchell, full case report, 'Doctors' Association UK,' 1 December 2021 *<https://dauk.org/Toombes-v-Mitchell-Approved-Judgment.pdf>.*

83 E. Mahase, 'Doctors express "grave concerns" at GMC action after GP is suspended over laptop claim', *British Medical Journal* (2022), 377: 1324 *<www.bmj.com/content/377/bmj.o1324?ijkey=1aa3c1a476195b35dd6a666a71729f5397a09ded&keytype=tf_ipsecsha>.*

84 'GMC publishes report on deaths during investigations', GMC, 3 March 2022 <*www.gmc-uk.org/news/news-archive/gmc-publishes-report-on-deaths-during-investigations*>.

85 'GMC targets elimination of disproportionate complaints and training inequalities', GMC, 18 May 2021 <*www.gmc-uk.org/news/news-archive/gmc-targets-elimination-of-disproportionate-complaints-and-training-inequalities*>.

86 'Co-chairs of Dr Arora case review publish findings', GMC, 2 November 2022 <*www.gmc-uk.org/news/news-archive/co-chairs-of-dr-arora-case-review-publish-findings*>.

87 L. Toberty, 'It is so tiring trying to help patients who deserve better', *The Times*, 23 September 2022 <*www.thetimes.co.uk/article/it-is-so-tiring-trying-to-help-patients-who-deserve-better-mpfs95290*>.

88 S. Mitchell et al., 'GP home visits: essential patient care or disposable relic?', *British Journal of General Practice* (2020), 70 (695): 306–307 <*https://bjgp.org/content/70/695/306*>.

89 'Home Visits', Midland Health <*https://midlandhealth.co.uk/gp-consultation/acute-illness/home-visits/*>.

90 S. Mitchell et al., *British Journal of General Practice* (2020).

91 E. Welch, 'Don't bash remote GPs: we provide a valuable service', *The Times*, 2 December 2022 <*www.thetimes.co.uk/article/dont-bash-remote-gps-we-provide-a-valuable-service-368ckg3z5*>.

92 'How has technology changed – and changed us in the last 20 Years', World Economics Forum, 18 November 2020 <*www.weforum.org/agenda/2020/11/heres-how-technology-has-changed-and-changed-us-over-the-past-20-years/*>.

93 H. Salisbury, 'What happened to the video revolution?' *British Medical Journal* (2023), 382: 1706 <*www.bmj.com/content/382/bmj.p1706*>.

94 'Appointments in General Practice', 'NHS Digital' <*https://digital.nhs.uk/data-and-information/publications/statistical/appointments-in-general-practice#latest-statistics*>.

95 N. Bostock, 'GP Bank helps practices plug long-standing workforce gaps with remote consultations', GPonline (2023) <*www.gponline.com/gp-bank-helps-practices-plug-long-standing-workforce-gaps-remote-consultations/article/1829272*>.

96 P. Evans, 'GPs like me should only be expected to work from 9 to 5', metro.co.uk, 20 December 2022 <*https://metro.co.uk/2022/12/20/gps-like-me-should-only-be-expected-to-work-from-9-to-5-17961887/*>.

97 C. Tilley, 'Jeremy Hunt: I'm completely responsible for failure to boost GP workforce', Pulse, 29 April 2022 <*www.pulsetoday.co.uk/news/breaking-news/jeremy-hunt-im-completely-responsible-for-failure-to-boost-gp-workforce/*>.

98 'England GP representatives vote to cut core hours to 9am–5pm', Pulse, 24 November 2022 <*www.pulsetoday.co.uk/news/breaking-news/england-gp-representatives-vote-to-cut-core-hours-to-9am-5pm/*>.

99 'GPs vote to ballot for industrial action if "disastrous" contract changes are not renegotiated', BMA, 27 April 2023 <*www.bma.org.uk/bma-media-centre/*

gps-vote-to-ballot-for-industrial-action-if-disastrous-contract-changes-are-not-renegotiated>.

100 'Fact sheet for media and public on junior doctors' industrial action in England', BMA <www.bma.org.uk/media/6882/bma-ia-juniors-fact-sheet-for-journalists.pdf>.

101 'BMA announces longest strike by junior doctors in NHS history', BMA, 23 June 2023 <www.bma.org.uk/bma-media-centre/bma-announces-longest-strike-by-junior-doctors-in-nhs-history>.

102 P. Morland, *A Fortunate Woman* (London: Picador, 2022).

103 'GP Earnings and Expenses Estimates', NHS Digital, 1 September 2022 <https://digital.nhs.uk/data-and-information/publications/statistical/gp-earnings-and-expenses-estimates/2020-21#summary>.

104 'The state of medical education and practice in the UK: The workforce report 2022', GMC (2022) <www.gmc-uk.org/-/media/documents/workforce-report-2022---full-report_pdf-94540077.pdf>.

105 'Four in ten junior doctors plan to leave the NHS as soon as they can find another job, BMA council chair reveals in New Year's message', BMA, 29 December 2022 <www.bma.org.uk/bma-media-centre/four-in-ten-junior-doctors-plan-to-leave-the-nhs-as-soon-as-they-can-find-another-job-bma-council-chair-reveals-in-new-years-message-to-the-country>.

106 'The UK's Health-Care Breakdown Demands Radical Thinking', *The Washington Post*, 2 August 2023 <www.washingtonpost.com/business/2023/08/02/britain-s-nhs-crisis-demands-radical-thinking/5dbe8d84-30ed-11ee-85dd-5c3c97d6acda_story.html>.

107 N. Barnard, 'As an NHS doctor, I'm undervalued and overworked – so I'm moving abroad', metro.co.uk, 15 July 2022 <https://metro.co.uk/2022/07/15/as-an-nhs-doctor-im-undervalued-and-overworked-so-im-moving-abroad-16962133/>.

108 'Pay scales for consultants in England', BMA, 1 July 2023 <www.bma.org.uk/pay-and-contracts/pay/consultants-pay-scales/pay-scales-for-consultants-in-england>.

109 S. Jones et al., 'Association between delays to patient admission from the emergency department and all-cause 30-day mortality', *Emerg Med JJ* (2022), 39: 168–173 <https://emj.bmj.com/content/39/3/168>.

110 'Ambulance handover delays', Nuffield Trust, 27 April 2023 <www.nuffieldtrust.org.uk/resource/ambulance-handover-delays>.

111 'Mirror, mirror 2021: Reflecting poorly: Healthcare in the US compared to other high income countries', The Commonwealth Fund, 4 August 2021 <www.commonwealthfund.org/publications/fund-reports/2021/aug/mirror-mirror-2021-reflecting-poorly>.

112 The Norwegian Ministry of Health, 13 December 2022 <www.regjeringen.no/no/tema/helse-og-omsorg/helse--og-omsorgstjenester-i-kommunene/innsikt/fastlegeordningen/id115301/>.

113 I. K. Rebnord et al., 'Fastlegers tidsbruk', Bergen: Nasjonalt

kompetansesenter for legevaktmedisin, Uni Research Helse, 2018.

114 Helsedirektoratet (2019), Fastlegestatistikk [nettdokument], Oslo: Helsedirektoratet (lest 26. Desember 2022). Tilgjengelig fra *<www. helsedirektoratet.no/statistikk/fastlegestatistikk>*.

115 Norwegian regulation on providing GPs in Municipalities, Forskrift om fastlegeordning i kommunene, FOR-2012-08-29-842 *<https://lovdata.no/ dokument/SF/forskrift/2012-08-29-842>*.

116 GP-Crisis, The Norwegian Medical Association, December 2022 *<www. legeforeningen.no/foreningsledd/yf/allmennlegeforeningen/krisen-i-fastlegeordnin- gen/>*.

117 National government appoints expert committee, 11 August 2022 *<www.reg- jeringen.no/no/aktuelt/ekspertutvalg-skal-gjennomgå-fastlegeordningen/id2923958/>*.

118 I. Heath, 'The mystery of general practice', Nuffield Provincial Hospitals Trust, London (1995) *<www.nuffieldtrust.org.uk/sites/default/files/2017-01/the- mystery-of-general-practice-web-final.pdf>*.

119 'Visiting a doctor or nurse', Ministry for Health, updated 30 June 2022 *<www.health.govt.nz/your-health/services-and-support/health-care-services/visit- ing-doctor-or-nurse>*.

120 'Changes to the Medicines Regulations – what you need to know', March 2011, revised 25 October 2013 *<www.medsafe.govt.nz/profs/PUArticles/ChangestoMedi- cinesRegulations.htm>*.

121 PHARMAC, New Zealand Government *<https://pharmac.govt.nz/about/>*.

122 Prescription Subsidy Scheme, Ministry of Health, updated 2 June 2021 *<www.health.govt.nz/your-health/conditions-and-treatments/treatments-and-sur- gery/medications/prescription-subsidy-scheme>*.

123 'NHS prescription charges', NHS Services *<www.nhs.uk/nhs-services/pre- scriptions-and-pharmacies/nhs-prescription-charges/>*.

124 'Visiting a doctor or nurse', Ministry for Health, updated 30 June 2022

125 'Improving New Zealand's Quality of Life', ACC Prevention Care Recovery *<www.acc.co.nz>*.

126 H. Kluge, 'Statement – Strengthening health systems in Europe', European Public Health Conference, 2022, 10 November 2022 *<www.who.int/europe/news/ item/11-11-2022-statement---strengthening-health-systems-in-europe>*.

127 'BMA urges public to be kind as survey reveals worrying levels of abuse against doctors and colleagues', BMA Media Team, 10 August 2021 *<www.bma.org.uk/ bma-media-centre/bma-urges-public-to-be-kind-as-survey-reveals-worrying-levels- of-abuse-against-doctors-and-colleagues>*.

128 'GPs are being blamed for government failures in primary care, say doctors', *British Medical Journal* (2021), 372: n2234 *<https://doi.org/10.1136/bmj.n2234>*.

129 E. Bower, 'GP suicide sparks calls for measures to protect doctors from spiralling workloads', GPonline, 5 August 2022 *<www.gponline.com/gp-suicide- sparks-calls-measures-protect-doctors-spiralling-workloads/article/1795152>*.

130 'Guidance on Requirements for Registering with a GP – Standard Operating

Principles for Primary Medical Care', Wessex LMC (2022) *<www.wessexlmcs.com/patientregistration>*.

131 J. Kaffash and R. Carter, 'Revealed: The GP practices that have closed for good and why they have closed', Pulse, 29 August 2022 *<www.pulsetoday.co.uk/news/lost-practices/revealed-the-gp-practices-that-have-closed-for-good-and-why-they-have-closed/>*.

132 K. Bergman, 'Workload issues affecting GP trainees' plans for their future careers', The King's Fund, 7 September 2022 *<www.kingsfund.org.uk/blog/2022/09/workload-issues-affecting-gp-trainees-plans-for-their-future-careers>*.

133 '60% of GP training places remain unfilled in areas of England', Pulse, 28 April 2017 *<www.pulsetoday.co.uk/news/workforce/60-of-gp-training-places-remain-un-filled-in-areas-of-england/>*.

134 R. Carter, 'High vacancy rates persist as one in six GP positions unfilled', Pulse, 30 June 2022 *<www.pulsetoday.co.uk/news/workforce/high-vacancy-rates-persist-as-one-in-six-gp-positions-unfilled/>*.

135 A. Hodkinson et al., 'Associations of physician burnout with career engagement and quality of patient care: systematic review and meta-analysis', *British Medical Journal* (2022), 378: e070442 *<www.bmj.com/content/378/bmj-2022-070442>*.

136 'Safe Working in General Practice', BMA GPCE Committee, 10 November 2022 *<www.bma.org.uk/advice-and-support/gp-practices/managing-workload/safe-working-in-general-practice>*.

137 L. Haynes and N. Bostock, 'GP patient contacts running 84% above safe limit, poll suggests', GPonline, 25 January 2022 *<www.gponline.com/gp-patient-contacts-running-84-above-safe-limit-poll-suggests/article/1738032>*.

138 'Urgent action needed to reverse "mass exodus" of almost 19,000 GPs over the next five years, warns Royal College of GPs', Royal College of General Practitioners, 22 June 2022 *<www.rcgp.org.uk/News/Mass-exodus>*.

139 R. Murray, 'Demand and activity in the NHS: Still rising', The King's Fund, 21 December 2016 *<www.kingsfund.org.uk/blog/2016/12/demand-and-activi-ty-nhs-still-rising>*.

140 C. Baker, 'NHS pressures in England: Waiting times, demand and capac-ity', UK Parliament House of Commons Library, 17 December 2019 *<https://commonslibrary.parliament.uk/nhs-pressures-in-england-waiting-times-demand-and-capacity/>*.

141 S. Cattan et al., 'The health impacts of Sure Start', Institute for Fiscal Studies, 16 August 2021 *<https://ifs.org.uk/sites/default/files/output_url_files/BN332-The-health-impacts-of-sure-start-1.pdf>*,

142 S. Coughlan, 'Sure Start centres "big benefit" but face cuts', BBC News, 4 June 2019 *<www.bbc.co.uk/news/education-48498763>*.

143 'Specialist applications and certificates statistics', GMC *<www.gmc-uk.org/about/what-we-do-and-why/data-and-research/medical-practice-statistics-and-re-ports/specialist-applications-and-certificates>*.

144 'Induction and refresher scheme', Health Education England, NHS *<www.hee.*

nhs.uk/our-work/induction-refresher-scheme>.

145 N. Bostock, 'GPs per patient slump as NHS medical workforce "25 years behind EU", BMA warns', GPonline, 12 July 2021 *<www.gponline.com/gps-per-patient-slump-nhs-medical-workforce-25-years-behind-eu-bma-warns/article/1721892>.*

146 'Social determinants of health', World Health Organization *<www.who.int/health-topics/social-determinants-of-health#tab=tab_1>.*

147 S. Perry, 'Cuts to public health run counter to levelling up, say leading organisations', The Health Foundation, 5 October 2021 *<www.health.org.uk/news-and-comment/news/cuts-to-public-health-run-counter-to-levelling-up-say-leading-health-organisations>.*

148 L. Allen, 'Why cutting spending on public health is a false economy', University of Oxford Research *<www.ox.ac.uk/research/why-cutting-spending-public-health-false-economy>.*

149 'Public Health funding in England: Death by a thousand cuts', The Lancet Gastroenterology & Hepatology, 6(12); 971, 1 December 2021 *<https://doi.org/10.1016/S2468-1253(21)00394-0>.*

150 R. Kelly Crace and D. Brown, 'Life values inventory' *<www.lifevaluesinventory.org>.*

151 'GPs' working conditions are "lonely" and "damage" patient relationship, warns GMC', Pulse, 15 November 2019 *<www.pulsetoday.co.uk/news/regulation/gps-working-conditions-are-lonely-and-damage-patient-relationship-warns-gmc/>.*

152 J. Napier, 'Wellbeing for GPs: How can you find the "wiggle-room" to tackle stress?', GPonline, 14 April 2016 *<www.gponline.com/wellbeing-gps-find-wiggle-room-tackle-stress/article/1389717>.*

153 J. Napier, 'Preventing burnout for GPs: time is of the essence', 18 May 2016 *<www.linkedin.com/pulse/preventing-burnout-gps-time-essence-jennifer-napier>.*

154 B. Baird et al., 'Innovative models of general practice', The King's Fund, June 2018, 20–5 *<www.kingsfund.org.uk/projects/innovative-models-care-delivery-general-practice>.*

155 S. T. Iqbal and B. P. Bailey, 'Effects of intelligent notification management on users and their tasks', CHI (2008), 93–102 *<www.scinapse.io/papers/2087759743>.*

156 S. Gould et al., 'What does it mean for an interruption to be relevant? An investigation of relevance as a memory effect', Proceedings of the Human Factors and Ergonomics Society Annual Meeting, September 2013, 57(1): 149–153 *<http://dx.doi.org/10.1177/1541931213571034>.*

157 E. Woods, 'Health Care Costs Number One Cause of Bankruptcy for American Families', American Bankruptcy Institute *<www.abi.org/feed-item/health-care-costs-number-one-cause-of-bankruptcy-for-american-families>.*

158 E. Welch, 'I'm a GP – if Sajid Javid thinks charging patients will help us, he's wrong', metro.co.uk, 24 January 2023 *<https://metro.co.uk/2023/01/24/im-a-gp-if-sajid-javid-thinks-charging-patients-will-help-us-hes-wrong-18158360/>.*

159 Sajid Javid, 'We need to agree a new NHS future or 1948 dream dies', The

Times, 20 January 2023 <*www.thetimes.co.uk/article/sajid-javid-times-health-commission-we-need-to-agree-a-new-nhs-future-or-1948-dream-dies-2qp28b7d5*>.

160 D. O'Reilly et al., 'Consultation charges in Ireland deter a large proportion of patients from seeing the GP: Results of a cross-sectional survey', *Eur JJ Gen Pract* (2007), 13 (4): 231-6 <*https://pubmed.ncbi.nlm.nih.gov/18324505/*>.

161 'Sajid Javid calls for patients to pay for GP and A&E visits', *Guardian*, 20 January 2023 <*www.theguardian.com/politics/2023/jan/20/sajid-javid-calls-for-patients-to-pay-for-gp-and-ae-visits*>.

162 P. Tammes et al., 'Is continuity of primary care declining in England? Practice-level longitudinal study from 2012 to 2017', *British Journal of General Practice* (2021), 71 (707): e432-e440 <*https://bjgp.org/content/71/707/e432*>.

163 'Health at a glance', OECD, 2021 <*www.oecd-ilibrary.org/social-issues-migration-health/health-at-a-glance-2021_ae3016b9-en;jsessionid=dheFhgX25I-8GIp0dFzhIa8h37D1LxIrSAEXmfOIo.ip-10-240-5-70*>.

164 'Investment in general practice', BMA, 24 March 2022 <*www.bma.org.uk/advice-and-support/nhs-delivery-and-workforce/funding/investment-in-general-practice*>.

165 C. Potter, 'Record 4,032 doctors to start GP training placements by February', Pulse, 23 November 2022 <*www.pulsetoday.co.uk/news/education-and-training/record-4032-doctors-to-start-gp-training-placements-by-february/*>.

166 '2023 GP Patient Survey', IPSOS, 13 July 2023 <*www.ipsos.com/en-uk/2023-gp-patient-survey-results-released*>.

167 B. Starfield et al., 'Contribution of primary care to health systems and health', *The Milbank Quarterly*, 3 October 2005 <*www.pubmed.ncbi.nlm.nih.gov/16202000*>.

168 S. Basu et al., 'Association of primary care physician supply with population mortality in the United States, 2005–2015', *JAMA Intern Med*, 18 February 2019 <*https://jamanetwork.com/journals/jamainternalmedicine/fullarticle/2724393*>.

169 'Study shows impact of high GP turnover on service and health', University of Manchester, 24 January 2023 <*www.manchester.ac.uk/discover/news/study-shows-impact-of-high-gp-turnover-on-service-and-health/*>.

170 H. Sandvik, 'Continuity in general practice as predictor of mortality, acute hospitalisation, and use of out-of-hours care: a registry-based observational study in Norway', *British Journal of General Practice* (2022), 72 (715): e84-e90 <*https://bjgp.org/content/72/715/e84*>.

171 S. Hodes, 'Primary care networks: More effort is needed to engage with general practices, says report', *British Medical Journal*, 20 November 2020, 371: <*www.bmj.com/content/371/bmj.m4551/rr*>.

172 'Clinical pharmacists vital to patient care in five year plan', NHSE, 31 January 2019 <*www.england.nhs.uk/2019/01/clinical-pharmacists-vital-to-patient-care-in-five-year-gp*>.

173 'Plans to bolster patient safety and boost support for frontline staff by

streamlining the system for healthcare regulators', Department of Health and Social Care, 18 February 2023 *<www.gov.uk/government/news/plans-to-bolster-patient-safety-and-boost-support-for-frontline-staff-by-streamlining-the-system-for-healthcare-regulators>*.

174 'All Wales Physician Governance Framework', NHS Wales *<https://heiw.nhs.wales/files/weds-designing-and-redesigning-physician-framework/all-wales-physician-associate-governance-framework/>*.

175 General Medical Council: PA and AA regulations *<www.gmc-uk.org/pa-and-aa-regulation-hub>*.

176 E. Dean, 'Physician associates in the media spotlight: what's the latest on the role?' *British Medical Journal* (2023), 382:1731 *<www.bmj.com/content/382/bmj.p1731>*.

177 M. Larkin, 'TAVI Turmoil: Did an ANP Perform Transcatheter Aortic Valve Replacement in the UK?', Medscape, 28 June 2023 *<www.medscape.com/viewarticle/993871>*.

178 A. Colivicchi, 'GP practice stops employing physicians associates after patient death', Pulse, 7 July 2023 *<www.pulsetoday.co.uk/news/clinical-areas/cardiovascular/gp-practice-stops-employing-physician-associates-after-patient-death/>*.

179 'DAUK urges GMC reevaluation: More than 2,800 doctors warn against PA regulation risks', Doctors' Association UK, 31 October 2023 *<www.dauk.org/news/2023/10/31/dauk-urges-gmc-reevaluation-over-2800-doctors-warn-against-pa-regulation-risks/>*

180 'BMA calls for immediate pause on recruitment of physician associates', *British Medical Journal*, 16 November 2023 *<www.bma.org.uk/bma-media-centre/bma-calls-for-immediate-pause-on-recruitment-of-physician-associates>*

181 'General Practice Workforce, 31 March 2022', NHS Digital, 28 April 2022 *<https://digital.nhs.uk/data-and-information/publications/statistical/general-and-personal-medical-services/31-march-2022>*.

182 B. N. Guest et al., 'Preparing physician associates to prescribe: evidence, educational frameworks and pathways', *Future Healthcare Journal*, March 2022 *<www.rcpjournals.org/content/futurehosp/9/1/21>*.

183 'Professionally Active Physicians', KFF *<www.kff.org/other/state-indicator/total-active-physicians/?currentTimeframe=0&selectedDistributions=specialist-physicians&sortModel=%7B%22colId%22:%22Location%22,%22sort%22:%22asc%22%7D>*.

184 'Occupational Employment and Wage Statistics', U. S. Bureau of Labor Statistics, May 2022 *<www.bls.gov/oes/current/oes291071.htm>*.

185 FPA Census *<www.fparcp.co.uk/about-fpa/fpa-census>*.

186 'The NHS Long Term Plan', NHS, 21 August 2019 *<www.longtermplan.nhs.uk/publication/nhs-long-term-plan/>*.

187 S. Hodes, 'Primary care networks: More effort is needed to engage with general practices, says report', *British Medical Journal*, 20 November 2020, 371:m4551 *<www.bmj.com/content/371/bmj.m4551/rr>*.

188 'At Your Service: A proposal to reform general practice and enable digital healthcare at scale', Policy Exchange, 4 March 2022 <*https://policyexchange.org. uk/publication/at-your-service/*>.

189 'Next steps for integrating primary care: Fuller stocktake report', NHS England, 26 May 2022 <*www.england.nhs.uk/publication/next-steps-for-integrating-primary-care-fuller-stocktake-report/*>.

190 E. Welch, 'Part-time GPs are not to blame for the downfall of the NHS right now', metro.co.uk, 26 April 2022 <*https://metro.co.uk/2022/04/26/part-time-gps-are-not-to-blame-for-the-downfall-of-the-nhs-right-now-16499208/*>.

191 S. Hodes et al., 'When part time means full time: the GP paradox', *British Medical Journal* (2022), 377 <*www.bmj.com/content/377/bmj.o1271*>.

192 '2023 GP Patient Survey', IPSOS (2023) <*www.ipsos.com/en-uk/2023-gp-patient-survey-results-released*>.

193 'General Practice Workforce, 30 November 2021', NHS Digital <*https:// digital.nhs.uk/data-and-information/publications/statistical/general-practice-workforce-archive/30-november-2021*>.

194 'Changing hours of work', BMA, 20 July 2021 <*www.bma.org.uk/pay-and-contracts/contracts/salaried-gp-contract/salaried-gp-model-contract-toolkit/changing-hours-of-work*>.

195 '2023 GP Patient Survey', IPSOS (2023).

196 'It is no longer feasible to be a full time GP', *The Sunday Times*, 24 July 2022, posted on X (formerly Twitter) <*https://twitter.com/hendopolis/status/1550952106718273540*>.

197 J. Kaffash, 'The "part time" fallacy', Pulse, 27 July 2022 <*www.pulsetoday. co.uk/views/editors-blog/the-part-time-fallacy*>.

198 'GMC supports call to recognise GPs as specialists', General Medical Council, 17 September 2019 <*www.gmc-uk.org/news/news-archive/gmc-supports-calls-to-recognise-gps-as-specialists*>.

199 'Learn Not Blame', Doctors' Association UK <*www.dauk.org/learnnotblame/*>.

200 'Nurse Lucy Letby guilty of murdering seven babies at Chester hospital', *Guardian*, 18 August 2023 <*www.theguardian.com/uk-news/2023/aug/18/lucy-letby-found-guilty-of-murdering-seven-babies-at-chester-hospital*>.

201 'Press Release: DAUK call for regulation of healthcare managers to improve accountability', Doctors' Association UK <*www.dauk.org/news/2023/08/24/ press-release-dauk-call-for-regulation-of-healthcare-managers-to-improve-accountability/*>.

202 H. Cole, 'Doc Won't See You', *Sun*, 23 July 2023 <*www.thesun.co.uk/ health/23150820/figures-two-week-wait-gp-appointments-england-nhs-crisis/*>.

203 'The Bawa-Garba case', *British Medical Journal* <*www.bmj.com/bawa-garba*>.

204 C. Potter, 'GPs demand IPSO investigation after Mail claims A&E crisis is "fuelled by GPs"', Pulse ,10 June 2022 <*www.pulsetoday.co.uk/news/urgent-care/ gps-demand-ipso-investigation-after-mail-claims-ae-crisis-is-fuelled-by-gps/*>.

About the Author

Dr Ellen Welch is a practising NHS GP, mum and co-chair of the Doctors' Association UK (DAUK) for 2022–3. Now based in Cumbria, she has worked in various roles within the NHS and around the world over the last 20 years including as a ski field doctor in New Zealand, an expedition medic in Tanzania and a cruise ship doctor in every continent except Antarctica. She has won awards at both the BMA and MJA annual awards for her previous publications. She is the author of *How the NHS Coped with Covid-19* (2022), *The NHS: The Story So Far* (2021) and *The NHS at 70: A Living History* (2018). She has written for *The Guardian, The Independent, The Times, Metro, GP Online* and the *British Medical Journal* among others. All royalties for this book will go to DAUK.